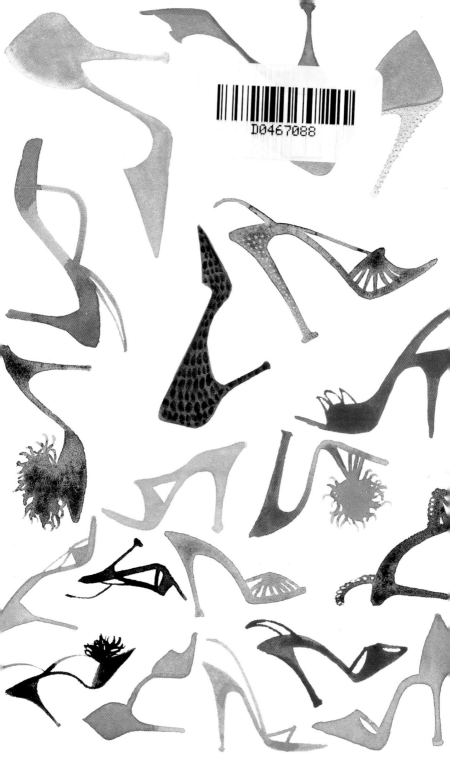

"Stover, Forrest and their colleagues are not only shrewd and insightfully observant field anthropologists, you sense that they would be personally adept at putting false eyelashes on a monkey."

—TOM ROBBINS

"The perfect little book for anyone who wants to fulfill her own Bombshell aspirations. Just grab your favorite baby doll pajamas, a glass of champagne, and sink right in!"

—MARISA TOMEI

"With prose and perception of rare and natural grace, Laren Stover, in this lilting *livre du blondisme*, has given us, modestly and unassumingly and sublimely, a work that deserves a place beside Neumann's *The Great Mother*, Witt's *Isis in the Ancient World*, and the complete run of *Beauty Parade*."

—NICK TOSCHES

"Ten, nine, eight, seven…get ready to detonate! The Bombshell girls have figured out the secret formula: how to mix equal parts lady and tramp. Consider this your literary compact. Slip it in your purse, balance it on your head, just keep it on hand—and refer to it as often as you touch up your lipstick. Kaboom!"

—ILENE ROSENZWEIG

THE

Bombshell

MANUAL OF STYLE

THE
Bombshell
MANUAL OF STYLE

LAREN STOVER **and** KIMBERLY FORREST

with Nicole Burdette and Randi Gollin

Illustrations by Ruben Toledo

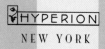

HYPERION

NEW YORK

Copyright © 2001 Laren Stover
Illustrations © 2001 Ruben Toledo

Library of Congress Cataloging-in-Publication Data

Stover, Laren.
The bombshell manual of style / Laren Stover and
Kimberly Forrest ; with Nicole Burdette and Randi Gollin ;
illustrations by Ruben Toledo.
p.   cm.
ISBN 0-7868-6694-2
1. Clothing and dress.   2. Fashion.
I. Forrest, Kimberly.   II. Title.

TT507.S855 2001
646'.34—dc21   00–059793

Design by Ruth Lee

FIRST EDITION

3   5   7   9   10   8   6   4

FOR

Christina Cooley

CONTENTS

III. BOMBSHELL LIFESTYLE

IV. BOMBSHELL PURSUITS & IDEALS

V. BOMBSHELL MISCELLANEA

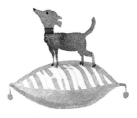

INTRODUCTION

When I told a friend I was working on a book about Bombshells, he said that all little girls grow up wanting to be either a sex kitten or a nun. I explained that to little girls, *The Song of Bernadette* was just as appealing as *Gentlemen Prefer Blondes*. That little girls want to be both.

My own Bombshell aspirations got off to a healthy start in fourth grade, before my mother squished them under her prim pump. My grandmother, a southern belle, gave me Lanvin's My Sin and my first stockings and high heels in aqua blue brocade. I practiced sashaying over the uneven brick path in her backyard in Baltimore, repeating my Bombshell mantra, "Why don't you come up and see me sometime." My grandmother also administered other, less wholesome, but nonetheless legendary Bombshell products—sleeping pills and smelling salts—something I've yet to tell my mother.

Mae West was my personal favorite for the throaty, controlling power she seemed to have over men. Marilyn Monroe, whom I adored for her naïveté and overt friendliness, was not highly regarded in my house; my mother, a serious thespian, declared Monroe was simply a body, not a talent, and worse, seemed to enjoy being ogled. So these trappings administered tenderly by my grandmother over the summers—in tandem with advice like "Men like polka dots"—were taboo at home.

Somewhere along the line I'd become the librarian type in oxfords. I lost the perspective I'd had as an aqua blue, high-heeled child; I'd forgotten that being a Bombshell is a state of mind.

My inner Bombshell was all but extinguished and I was leading a smart, sensible life enhanced by a little lipstick and an occasional rhinestone when I met a breathy, voluptuous blonde. She swished into morning meetings with Veronica Lake hair. She wore tight sweaters and 4-inch heels. She is the kind of woman who crosses the street without looking, Lady Dior handbag in hand (never a shoulder strap). She's the kind of woman who has pictures of herself cuddling pets and makes donations to the American Anti-Vivisection Society, but wishes they wouldn't send those gruesome pictures. She is a lush landscape, and her smile is an invitation to enjoy the view. But I didn't end up in her thrall until the day I threw a grammar question out to the room and she was the only one who responded. "Don't you have *The Chicago Manual of Style*?" she asked in her sultry tone. "Here, borrow mine."

It was then that I realized a Bombshell could be brainy. Later I discovered it might even be a prerequisite. The Bombshell is as complex as she is compelling. She is both provocative and misunderstood, a sort of endangered species. I decided right then and there to write *The Bombshell Manual of Style*. It would be a comprehensive book with all the ingredients that make a Bombshell tick, from her shoes to her favorite writers. At first I felt shy telling people about this project. It seemed so un-PC. But my women friends acted like I'd just uncorked a bottle of vintage Dom Pérignon. Men (especially men) said they were dying to read it when it came out. My friends had lots to say about Bombshells—unexpected, witty, reverent things that seemed to ring true. I decided the book would have greater breadth and depth with the nuances of a collective mind.

My collaborators on this project are some of the most intelligent writers I know. They were craving a subject that was smart but scintillating. They wanted to dot their *i*'s with sequins, construct paragraphs in lamé, script headlines in marabou. They wanted to wiggle, stride or sashay (their personal choice) across a room in mules. Or watch a Bombshell do all of the above. They wanted to see Jayne Mansfield coo in a bubble bath, Dorothy Dandridge steam things up, Ava Gardner kick off her shoes.

Everyone involved has a different area of expertise. Kimberly Forrest wrote and edited the book with me— perched on a chair in my apartment, or curled on a couch at our Woodstock getaway. She used a pink highlighter and ordered in champagne. Nicole Burdette had an unfair advantage, having grown up with a Bombshell mom. Her knowledge of Bombshells is both empirical and instinctive. She knew what shoes Brigitte Bardot wore in every film, all of Marilyn Monroe's rhinestone placements and had a sixth sense about what the Bombshell does and does not read. Many of Nicole's library suggestions were substantiated when Christie's put Marilyn Monroe's book collection on display. Randi Gollin, who spent months at various libraries, knew the right music for every Bombshell mood and rattled off the Bombshell's favorite films in a heartbeat. She's rather private but I suspect she's gone out and purchased a pair of marabou mules.

We held a few Bombshell roundtables and concurred on the following points: that this iconic creature is as vulnerable as she is glamorous. That she seeks to give pleasure, and is never a gold digger. That the Bombshell is concerned with social protocol, and even when she has a job that exploits her Bombshell figure, she is never trashy, trampy or a vamp. That a Bombshell has dignity, even if, and especially if, she's had a tragic childhood. We all agreed one of her favorite movies is *Bambi*. After reading about real Bombshell lives, our respect for her deepened. The Bombshell proves you don't need to have privilege to triumph, to be buoyant or to be beautiful.

Christie's auction of the personal property of Marilyn Monroe confirmed many of our Bombshell maxims. Seeing Marilyn's books, her sad personal notes, her humble and sentimental everyday objects showed that a Bombshell is not, as legend dictates, devastatingly dumb, but devastatingly complex. A Bombshell is a woman who has learned to use her vulnerability to her advantage, a woman who allows for her frailty and breakable humanity, but does not let it eclipse her aura of glamour.

We did a reading of an early version of this book in the Helen Hayes Gallery at the Algonquin Hotel and among the readers was Academy Award-winning Bombshell Marisa Tomei, who read in a barely closed kimono and stilettos. In the Algonquin hotel room before the reading, Marisa looked over her text. "'The Bombshell refrigerator is a sort of vanity on ice . . .'" Turning to her friend she said, "That's mine, isn't it, Frank?"

LAREN STOVER
New York City, 2000

I

Bombshell Psychology

What Makes a Bombshell Tick

A Bombshell is full of contradictions. She is a combustible blend of confidence and vulnerability. Sauce and naïveté. She wears high heels but kicks them off at every opportunity. Adores negligées and charmeuse gowns but can't wait to get out of them. She always expects to run into someone who matters, even if she's home alone. A Bombshell never dresses carelessly and wears marabou mules around the house. She behaves as if all life's a movie in which she is the star.

A Bombshell Radiates Confidence

When she enters a room, everyone looks.[1] When she exits a room, everyone looks. Not because she is more beautiful than

---

1 Of Jayne Mansfield, a costar said, "She just walked out and assumed everyone would be interested in her, and therefore, we all were."

other women, or because her clothing is more ooh-la-la—
a Bombshell's magnetism flows from the inside out.[2]

A Bombshell is comfortable and familiar with her body.
She wants other people to feel comfortable with her, too.
She doesn't edit her feelings or her body language. She is, in
fact, extravagant with her body language. She touches people. Spontaneously.

She expresses her feelings as openly as she displays her
curves. Her body may be human and imperfect, not at all
mannequin-like, yet she puts herself on a pedestal as easily as
she lounges on a couch.

"She wasn't classically beautiful by any means," writes
W. J. Weatherby in his book, *Conversations with Marilyn*, "but
she had a strong, attractive body and chameleon moods that
could make her body convey anything she wished."

A Bombshell Believes in
Her Fantasies

Even if her bracelet is dime-store cheap, she wears it as
though it were Cartier. She doesn't need real diamonds to
feel like a million dollars. She knows they'll come in good
time. She expects people to send flowers and stop by with
champagne. And somehow, they do. Watching her emote
over a bouquet is a performance that her suitors and fans
want to see again and again.[3] She dreams in French, some-

2 "Sex appeal," said Dorothy Dandridge, "doesn't depend entirely on
physical attributes; it's a kind of vitality and energy, a—well, an undercur-
rent of vitality. It has to do with how you feel as a person."

3 Richard Burton once said, "The wonderful thing about Elizabeth {Taylor}
is that she loves jewels so much that she makes even a stingy man like me
want to give her jewelry just to see the thrill she gets when she sees it."

times Italian. She may have dropped out of her language class after two or three sessions, but she's seen enough foreign films to understand the languages of love.

A Bombshell Is Authentic

Some women cultivate a blasé attitude. They act bored. They think this makes them sophisticated. The Bombshell is never bored and, therefore, never boring. She never pretends to be anyone other than herself. She is not censored, careful or contrived. She doesn't read the rules or follow the rules, or color her hair to conform to the latest trend. The Bombshell cannot pretend excitement not deeply felt, nor gush over movies and books and art she finds disagreeable. She is not afraid of the truth, though she understands some lies—tiny lies—make life more effervescent. To a friend wearing a dress that is too tight, she might say, "You've lost weight!" but never, "You look fabulous!" The Bombshell has her own sense of ethics to which she is always true.

A Bombshell Is Vulnerable

While some women contrive to cover their hearts, the Bombshell reveals her feelings without calculating the consequences, regardless of the risk. She is so in tune with her emotions that she allows them to surface in a heartbeat. However, she is so endearing that most people are more inclined to come to her rescue than to do her harm. This is not southern belle helplessness she is affecting; she is expressing a genuine need to be loved. Her posture is always erect, her shoulders relaxed so that her chest is thrust forward, thus exposing her heart.

A Bombshell Is Resilient

Bombshells prove you don't need to have an enchanted childhood[4] or privilege to triumph. Failure—a film that bombs, a job that doesn't pan out, a marriage on the rocks, an unpublishable manuscript—is only a mild setback, and will at least garner some sort of publicity. (If there's a silver lining, the Bombshell always finds it.) No matter what's going on her in life, the Bombshell finds everyday occurrences thrilling.

A Bombshell Puts Glamour Before Comfort

A Bombshell is willing to overcome a little discomfort for a nude leg on a cold day. She doesn't complain that her feet hurt in 4-inch heels. She endures the constraints of boned underpinnings, and even celebrates them. It does not matter if anyone is going to see her garters. She wears them to please herself as much as to give pleasure to others. She dresses up for evenings at home with friends, even if it's just to watch the Academy Awards.

A Bombshell Is Compassionate

She always follows her heart. She wants to rescue animals. All animals. Lions, monkeys, kittens, beagles. She is too loving and innocent to be malicious. While she might have a

---

4 It's widely known that Marilyn Monroe spent her childhood in foster homes and that Dorothy Dandridge was routinely disciplined with a hairbrush.

temper—one of her charms—she never plots. She is a good listener. (She cries if you cry, then she'll try to cheer you up.) She is the kind of person others can't wait to share their news with because she is genuinely interested and effusive. She embraces the human condition while always adding a little glitter.

A Bombshell Is Intelligent

Her awe and wonder are sometimes construed as naïveté. She's smart enough to know that it doesn't matter if other people think she's too sensual or pretty to be brainy. She's never obnoxious or loud when she's right. She doesn't correct people. A Bombshell brushes up on topics that will enhance her social life. She does this not only because she has a genuine interest in everything, but because she wants others to feel comfortable. If she's going to have dinner with the director of the Museum of Modern Art and there's a Jackson Pollock show up, she'll reference her favorite painting with a comment like, "There really should be a perfume called Autumn Rhythm, don't you think?"

THINGS BOMBSHELLS GET AWAY WITH ORDINARY WOMEN CAN'T

Crying	*Over broken hearts, sad movies and nature films.*
Flirting	*With both men and women.*
Having no domestic prowess	*She doesn't mastermind the home; she lounges in it. She beautifies in it. She orders in.*
Tantrums	*She breaks china and throws drinks in private and public.*
Never paying	*For drinks. Dinner. Or anything.*
Lying about lovers	*The names and numbers always vary.*
Showing up late, but not as late as divas	*She tries to be on time, she really does. But heels break, puppies slow her down and she can't resist picking up the phone if it rings when she's running out the door. Not stopping to talk to an elderly neighbor is unthinkable.*
Reckless attire	*A Bombshell is innocently inappropriate. She will go braless or wear stilettos and tight sweaters to office meetings. Seamed stockings and fishnets are also acceptable as are "rocks" for day, always strategically positioned.*
Petty crimes	*Not returning engagement rings (when she calls it off) or jewelry and couture gowns borrowed for public appearances.*

Bombshell Words
to Live By

"My approach to beauty begins not with the face or figure but with the mind. If you can learn to use your mind as well as you use a powder puff, you will become more truly beautiful."

—Sophia Loren

"The truth about beauty is if you always have it, you always know it."

—Kim Basinger

"I find that I regret nothing. There are three words I have never said, and never will. They are, 'I am sorry.'"

—Dolores Del Rio

"I am not difficult. I am definite."

—Hedy Lamarr

"The only thing I really believe in is love."

—Brigitte Bardot

"I've never known what it is I was supposed to have had. All I do know is that sex appeal isn't make-believe. It's not the way you look or the way you walk or the way you smile, it's the way you are."

—LANA TURNER

"I finally realized I don't have to have an A-plus perfect body, and now I'm very happy the way I am."

—DREW BARRYMORE

On being asked to be in the Columbus Day Parade: "What the world does not know about me is that I am very emotional. I may look calm and collected, but I am extremely emotional inside and I'm afraid that I may cry all the way up Fifth Avenue."

—SOPHIA LOREN

"So long as a woman has twinkles in her eyes, no man notices whether she has wrinkles under them."

—DOLORES DEL RIO

"Any woman can look her best if she feels good in her skin. It's not a question of clothes or makeup. It's how she sparkles."

—SOPHIA LOREN

"If you use your imagination, you can look at any actress and see her nude. I hope to make you use your imagination."

—HEDY LAMARR

"There must be thousands of girls sitting alone like me dreaming about becoming a movie star. But I'm not going to worry about them, because I'm dreaming the hardest."

—MARILYN MONROE

"Sex appeal is good—but not in bad taste. Then it's ugly. I don't think a star has any business posing in a vulgar way. I've seen plenty of pin-up pictures that have sex appeal, interest and allure, but they're not vulgar. They have a little art to them. Marilyn's {Monroe} calendar was artistic."

—Jane Russell

On doing a nude scene: "But then some woman in the movie theater is going to sit there and say, 'Well, my body doesn't look like that,' and compare herself to something that isn't really fair. So I said, 'Well, I'm not going to work out at all and I'm just going to eat candy and ice cream when I have to be naked.'"

—Patricia Arquette

"If a girl has curviness, exciting lips, and a certain breath-lessness, it helps. And it won't do a bit of harm if she also has a kittenish, soft and cuddly quality."

—Jayne Mansfield

"You don't start a movie expecting to crash. You get married expecting it to be forever. That's why you get married."

—Elizabeth Taylor

"With a figure like mine a girl is certain to attract atten-tion—and I find it pleasing and necessary that men look at me. But when they get too attentive I give them the Mansfield Routine A. I tell them how much I trust them and value their advice and friendship. This startles the wolfiest of wolves into submission and almost immedi-ately he becomes fatherly or even brotherly."

—Jayne Mansfield

"The two big advantages I had at birth were to have been born wise and to have been born in poverty."

—SOPHIA LOREN

"All I know about acting is, you just do it. God bless Stanislavsky, but I can't even pronounce his name."

—KIM BASINGER

When asked if she objected to being called a blonde Bombshell: "I feel like a woman, and a 'Bombshell,' as you call it, is a woman in crescendo."

—JAYNE MANSFIELD

"I've got plenty of time to daydream and I'd rather daydream than do anything in the world."

—JANE RUSSELL

"I'm a naturally lazy person . . . I'd rather put on a bathing suit and lie in the sun beside my pool than be energetic or athletic."

—JEAN HARLOW

"A lady should be able to look sophisticated in an elegant evening gown and blossom forth like a rosebud in a bikini."

— JAYNE MANSFIELD

"Everyone is like a butterfly, they start out ugly and awkward and then morph into beautiful, graceful butterflies that everyone loves."

—DREW BARRYMORE

About her role as a blonde: "It's time that the blonde glamour girl dropped her modern offhand manner and assumed the seductive ways of the traditional charmer. We should be dangerous characters. Just think of Garbo and Dietrich and Harlow—they were really dangerous. When they gave a man the come-hither look, the poor guy didn't know whether he was going to be kissed or killed."

—KIM NOVAK

"I don't think I am a beautiful woman. Ava Gardner is. I think Audrey Hepburn is. But the way I look is all right with me. Because I want to be me. I don't take vitamins or do exercise. I can lose weight when I want to, mainly by just not eating."

—ELIZABETH TAYLOR

"It's a shallow, inconsistent, competitive, cruel world. Whenever I get really sad that I'm involved in it, I feel that instead of sitting on the sidelines and complaining, I should go in there and make it better."

—DREW BARRYMORE

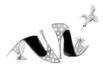

WHAT'S IN A NAME

A Bombshell is never named Phyllis, Edith or Bertha. And if she were you'd never know. Serious Bombshells take on names with va-va-voom, breathy alliteration and starlet potential. Names with marquee appeal.

Some Bombshells lift their names from a family member. Jean Harlow replaced four-syllable *Carpentier* with her mother's maiden name. A name that starts with a whispered exhalation, gets roped in with a lavish *l* and results in a pouty *o*, *Harlow* virtually conveys a platinum blonde lounging in ivory silk charmeuse. Marilyn Monroe, born Norma Jean Mortenson, took her last name from her grandmother and started from scratch with her first. Others simplify. Jane Russell dropped sincere, virtuous Ernestine for something simpler and let *Russell*, with its double curvy *s*'s, steal the show.

A Bombshell wants a name that will have a ripple effect, a name that resonates. It should go with her hair color. Never anything weird, slatternly, hard to pronounce, or with tawdry overtones. She also likes a name that looks good in an autograph. When it came time for Lana Turner to sign a contract she scrapped Julia Jean Mildred Frances Turner in favor of Lana. She couldn't resist that big, curvy *L*.

Unless she's a drag queen, she never takes another Bombshell's name. A Bombshell never walks in the shadow of a legend. She would not choose *Marilyn*, *Lana*, *Sophia*, *Brigitte* or *Ava*. And *Kim* is pushing it.

HOLLYWOOD BOMBSHELL NAME CHANGES

Brigitte Bardot	Camille Javal Bardot
Dolores Del Rio	Lolita Dolores Martinez Asunsolo Lopez Negrette
Jean Harlow	Harlean Carpentier
Rita Hayworth	Margarita Carmen Cansino
Veronica Lake	Constance Francis Ockleman
Dorothy Lamour	Mary Leta Dorothy Slaton
Sophia Loren	Sophia Villani Scicolone
Jayne Mansfield	Vera Jane Palmer
Marilyn Monroe	Norma Jean Mortenson
Kim Novak	Marilyn Pauline Novak
Jane Russell	Ernestine Jane Russell
Lana Turner	Julia Jean Mildred Frances Turner

BOMBSHELL
BODY LANGUAGE

Every movement counts. A Bombshell never thoughtlessly enters a room or flops into a chair. She has poise, good posture, va-va-voom. She's not afraid to *wow* the whole room. Dorothy Dandridge knew how. At one of her nightclub venues it was said she "came wriggling out of the wings like a caterpillar on a hot rock." The Bombshell has a way of making even the most rigid piece of furniture look comfortable.

Making an Entrance

The Bombshell understands the importance of the doorway. To the casual observer, it is the opening between two rooms; to the Bombshell it is the threshold between worlds, her launching pad. The Bombshell knows the doorway is the ultimate point of tension, one of architecture's power points. She does not calculate the amount of time she will linger here, but seems to intuit that how long she puts off her debut is in direct proportion to the effect she will have. An entire day/event/

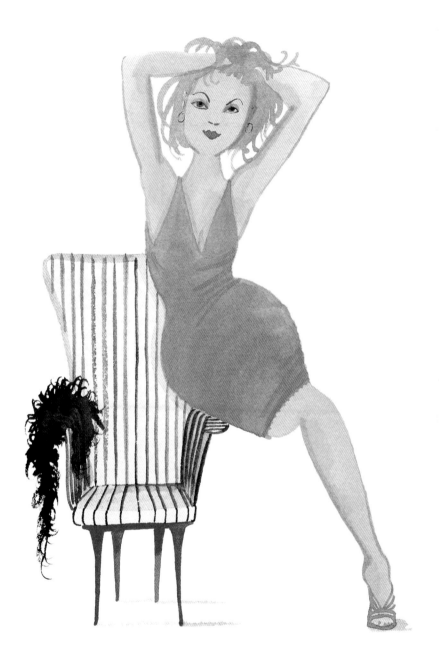

evening rests upon her ability to hold the room spellbound. A Bombshell always enters the room just before her audience gets antsy.

Lana Turner, in the original *The Postman Always Rings Twice*, makes her entrance, not at the top of a grand staircase, or into a ballroom, but in a simple doorway. She does not need to be wearing a ball gown or dramatic jewelry to create a sensation. Short shorts, a midriff top and heels will do.

She drops her lipstick and expects the man in question to pick it up while she assumes a goddesslike pose, legs in the graceful *contrapposto* position similar to Botticelli's *The Birth of Venus* and the *Medici Venus* sculpture. She puts all her weight on the left leg while bending the right, arching and pointing her foot. The top of her body is slightly turned away. She gazes into her compact and only looks up when the man has asked her if she's lost something. Her response involves inhalation. This enhances her bustline, which frankly, she does not mind.

Elizabeth Taylor lingers to perfection in *A Place in the Sun*. First, she nonchalantly walks past the billiard room as though she has not noticed her love interest,

Montgomery Clift, alone at the table. She returns, curls her fingers around the door and presses half her body against it with provocative hesitancy. After she has engaged his attention, she runs her hand along the door edge to heighten the tension. Will she come in? Or slip away? Once she's in, she takes the long route around the table to his side, running her hand along the polished wooden edge of the billiard table before touching a piece of candy, popping it in her mouth, rounding the final edge and posing between two paintings. Bombshells love a little framing around them.

Jayne Mansfield projects boldly from the threshold into a roomful of men in *Too Hot to Handle*. Her entrance is of the full-frontal variety: shoulders back, arms stretched out and bent at the elbows to lightly touch the door frame and the open door, causing her chest to thrust forward. Her objective, once she has lingered at the door, is to sashay across the room to sit on the arm of the chair of her love interest, but not before she pauses, hands on hips, in front of the man who has just commented, "Hey, that's a very nice dress you've nearly got on." A Bombshell believes the right move is worth a thousand words.

Deplaning

The Bombshell never underestimates shock value, but uses it with discretion. When a Bombshell is feeling her oats she may flash and go. This works best when deplaning directly onto the tarmac.

Jayne Mansfield demonstrates the ultimate deplaning in *Will Success Spoil Rock Hunter?* She exits with her coat closed, hood up, stops at the first step, opens her coat, takes a step down and waves—it is at this point that we realize all she is wearing under the coat is a one-piece bathing suit, very

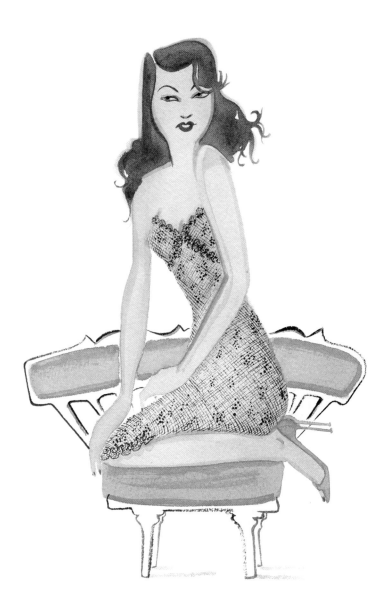

fancy. Her only other clothing: white high-heeled mules, long, white gloves and long rhinestone earrings. She blows kisses with both hands to her audience while allowing the wind to work her coat open. Once her kisses are returned, she descends. This works best on private planes.

The Audition/Interview

It's a tricky combination of bold and demure. A Bombshell always wears what she considers the appropriate clothing for the situation at hand. For a job interview or audition of a glamorous yet wholesome nature, she wears a fitted suit. The color will not be too sophisticated (taupe), severe (black), simmering (red), or lusty (leopard). When a Bombshell wants to appear nonthreatening and at the pinnacle of her femininity, pink is her color. Rhinestones always figure in somewhere. A Bombshell will hover at the threshold of the interviewer's office until she is greeted. She will smile and make eye contact until they are face to face. When asked to take a seat, the Bombshell will never sink into the chair offered if the interviewer is still standing, but will perch on the edge of the arm rest. When the interviewer sits down, the Bombshell will perch politely on the edge of her chair as if captivated, legs crossed at the ankles. See Rita Hayworth in *Cover Girl* for additional details.

Sitting

Bombshells don't sit exactly. They perch, curl, curve, and occasionally fling their legs up over the arm of the chair or back of the sofa. This also goes for seats on airplanes, cars and trains.

In *How to Marry a Millionaire*, Marilyn Monroe scoots

into a chair and curls kittenishly before answering the telephone. It doesn't matter that the person on the other end can't see her, her coquetry will radiate through the wires. Sofas and beds present a world of opportunity to the Bombshell. She may lie on her stomach propped up on her elbows with legs kicked into the air, curl around a pillow or pet, or lie on her back with legs bent. This is the position she prefers for reading and eating grapes.

Exits

The Bombshell exit doesn't start at the door. It's about getting there. Wiggling through chairs, spilling a little champagne, mesmerizing with an elegant arm gesture in an elbow-length glove, she makes herself noticed. Her outer garment—wrap, coat or scarf—will slip off her shoulders en route, insinuating a sort of chaos, and suggesting that she might just lose it all together. A Bombshell assumes everyone is interested.

If she's not in a huff—breaking vases, throwing glasses, leaving a trail of debris on the way to a grand door slam— she will, upon reaching the doorway, take a final glance over her shoulder, gazing out across the room as if taking in a beautiful landscape. On special occasions the Bombshell blows a kiss.

Bombshells also make dramatic exits from automobiles. They do this not by getting out quickly, but by swiveling gracefully toward the door and extending one leg with a languid movement and arched foot so that the toes hit the ground first. Bombshells always exit with an inhalation as if something wonderful is about to happen.

Bombshell Tantrums

The Bombshell is generally good natured. Although there are a few things that get to her—rudeness to waiters, under-tipping, married men who don't wear wedding rings, and nature films on public television ("How can the cameraman not do something?")—it is an insult to her pride that most frequently triggers a tantrum.

There are two types of Bombshell tantrums, blonde and brunette. The brunette kind is the one to watch out for. A blonde temper tantrum is a carefully orchestrated event, starting out with a surprised expression and a slight elevation of voice—never shrill but with powdery undertones. At this point she will do one of two things: stomp her foot, utter "How dare you," or "Well, I never," and fling her stole or wrap around, careful to slap the offending party across the face before sashaying out of the room; or, she will lift her champagne glass—a blonde Bombshell prefers to be drinking champagne when making a point—and splash the afore-mentioned party. She will also douse offenders with

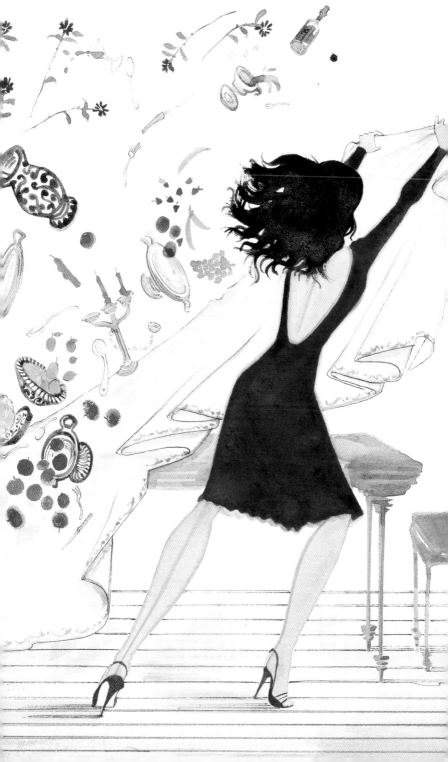

chardonnay, a martini, or any light or clear beverage, but never red wine as this she would consider vulgar.

The blonde Bombshell will also throw soft objects but is careful not to break lamps and china.

The brunette makes her point by smashing her glass against a wall, occasionally a window. Any other stemware within reach is considered fair game—vases, plates, anything breakable—no item is too precious for a brunette in a bad mood. Face creams, perfume bottles, shoes, even scissors, depending upon the severity of the offense. She has a sense of rhythm and will smash in sync to whatever music is on, preferably something jazzy although Tchaikovsky and Strauss also work.

Addendum: Redheads. Redhead tantrums are of the vocal variety, although Rita Hayworth in a rage is said to have broken all the windows of her beau's apartment by driving golf balls through them. It should be noted that Rita Hayworth's natural hair color was dark brown.

Bombshell Fashion
& Beauty

BOMBSHELL FASHION

The Bombshell takes her clothing personally. She'll pass on trends like baseball caps, even with sequins. The Bombshell knows a thing or two about anatomy and chooses outfits that accentuate her assets and amplify her personality. Nothing underwhelming or more enthusiastic than she is. She's not afraid to show up in scarlet when everyone's wearing the little black dress. That scarlet number will become the centerpiece of the room.

Bombshell clothing requires good posture: Fitted sweaters. Cinched waists. Tight skirts. Yet under no circumstances does the Bombshell wear clothing that could be construed as sleazy. She just wears her outfits a little tighter than the average woman,[1] even if she's meeting a queen. Whether it's low cut in the front or back or sliced to there, there is often a surprise peek of skin.

No matter how mundane the occasion, the Bombshell has an outfit in mind. She plays dress up every day.

---

1 The phrase *poured in* was coined in the thirties for Mae West.

Road-Tested Outfits
for Fifteen Occasions

1   *Poolside*   Shimmering white "girdle-front" one-piece bathing suit, 3-inch ankle-strap sandals, immense straw sun hat with ribbon tie. This is not worn on the head, but slung over the back and tied at the neck. (Inspiration: Dolores Del Rio photograph)

2   *Boxing Match*   Platinum sleeveless beaded gown with white stole. (Inspiration: Dorothy Dandridge in *Carmen Jones*)

3   *At the Easel*   White cotton French-cuffed shirt tucked into slim black trousers, black beret worn on a tilt, dangling pearl earrings. (Inspiration: Jayne Mansfield in *Panic Button*)

4   *South Seas Cruise*   Island-print sarong skirt knotted at hip with matching halter top embroidered with tiny shells, two banded cuffs—one on each wrist—crescent hoop earrings, black pumps and nylons, straw clutch and straw coolie hat worn on a tilt. (Inspiration: Jane Russell in *Macao*)

5   *Weight lifting at Home*   Denim jeans and triangle bikini top. (Inspiration: Marilyn Monroe photograph)

6   *Exercise Class with Personal Trainer*   White leotard. (Inspiration: Dorothy Dandridge photograph)

7   *Baby Shower*   Fitted, scoop-neck dress with cap sleeves in white with abstract floral motif, knee length with fishtail back and white 3-inch pumps. (Inspiration: Jayne Mansfield in *Promises! Promises!*)

8   *Acting Class*   Black unitard or turtleneck with slim black pants and black ballet slippers. (Inspiration: Jayne Mansfield in *Panic Button*)

9   *Movie Premiere*   Cerulean satin strapless gown with bead-encrusted bodice, sapphire and diamond necklace dripping into cleavage with matching dangling earrings, white gloves, white clutch, white stole. (Inspiration: Ava Gardner in *The Barefoot Contessa*)

10   *Motor Scooter Ride*   Burnt orange cotton dress with a mid-calf tiered, ruffled skirt and coordinating scarf tied under the chin. (Inspiration: Gina Lollobrigida, sidesaddle, in *Come September*)

11   *Diner*   Tight, periwinkle V-neck cashmere sweater with short sleeves, navy pencil skirt, silver necklace with small pearl or diamond pendant. (Inspiration: Kim Novak in *Pal Joey*)

12   *To the Office*   Skin-tight pale pink sweater unbuttoned to the fourth button, sleeves casually pushed up to the elbows and a knee-length pencil skirt in glen plaid. No bra evident. (Inspiration: Brigitte Bardot in *Une Parisienne*)

13   *Fancy Horseback Riding*   White cotton buttoned-up shirt with ruffles, black bolero jacket, gaucho hat and a full, long black skirt. (Inspiration: Rita Hayworth in *Blood and Sand*)

14   *Casual Horseback Riding*   Slim, plaid button-down shirt, elbow length, with cuffed jeans. Optional: bathing suit underneath. (Inspiration: Elizabeth Taylor in *A Place in the Sun*)

15   *Daytime Wear, City or Country*   The fitted, sometimes flounced black-and-white polka-dot dress. This item of clothing is essential to every Bombshell wardrobe. Polka dots are large, never tiny, Swiss or shy. It also comes in red-and-white. (Inspiration: Josephine Baker in *Zouzou*, Rita Hayworth in *Lady from Shanghai*, Marilyn Monroe in *The Misfits*)

Where the Bombshell Shops

The Bombshell likes exclusive stores and boutiques. She loves to go in and try things on.

A Bombshell favors a store with a reputation. Bombshell favorites are Ferragamo, Burberry, Christian Dior, Gucci, Henri Bendel (she adores the cozy cafe as well), Saks Fifth Avenue, Cartier and Tiffany to name a few. She has gone window-shopping at Fred Leighton, Harry Winston, Van Cleef & Arpels, Cartier and Tiffany, but generally buys her rhinestones at Zitomer on the Upper East Side in New York, Saks Fifth Avenue or at Gump's in San Francisco.

DESIGNERS FAVORED BY THE BOMBSHELL

Burberry (trench coats only)

William Calvert

Chloé

Christian Dior

Tracy Feith (when she's feeling very Carmen Jones)

Gucci

Levi's (jeans)

Marc Jacobs (when she's feeling girlish)

Marni

Pucci and vintage Pucci

Anna Sui

Yves St. Laurent

Valentino

THE ART OF SPARKLE, SHIMMER & SHINE

It goes way beyond "diamonds are a girl's best friend." This implies that the Bombshell is a gold digger. The true Bombshell is the opposite of the gold digger. The gold digger seeks pleasure. A free ride. Major carats. The Bombshell wants to give pleasure, to be loved, be adored and her rocks are an invitation to the view, i.e., her best locations. When she wears a rhinestone brooch at her cleavage, for example, she is simply allowing you to look at her chest.

A Bombshell might love Cartier, Tiffany, Harry Winston and Van Cleef & Arpels, but she knows rhinestones will do the trick. She is more concerned with effect than value. There is a famous Philippe Halsman photo of Marilyn Monroe in a white gathered dress with very little means of staying up; a glittering brooch at the cleavage is the centerpiece. We are not looking at her pondering the value of the stone. In fact, we could care less. That is how we know she is a Bombshell. With careful placement, the "diamond" brooch works wonders, even with no skin showing at all. In *Will Success Spoil Rock Hunter?*, Jayne Mansfield wears a high-necked dress with a strategically placed brooch that makes décolletage unnecessary.

It goes without saying that the proper attitude must accompany Bombshell rocks. The Bombshell cannot let her jewelry outshine her, her energy must live up to the glitter, surpass it even. She turns everything up a notch—her posture, her laughter (breathier, not louder), her highest heels. When drama is necessary, a Bombshell will choose a menagerie of "diamonds" so she will always be the center of attention. Bette Davis, outfitted by the incomparable Edith Head in one of her rare sexy roles—Margo Channing in *All About Eve*—wears a tight black dress with a big diamond brooch off to the side. Glittering earrings and bracelet further the admiration, allowing our eyes to race from wrist to neck to chest. Bombshell all the way.

Dangling earrings that sparkle are often favored by the Bombshell. They add radiance and draw light to her face. Dangling uninhibitedly, they suggest freedom by their movement and mirror her undulations. A small stud, regardless of its value, is always the last choice of the Bombshell. She'd rather let her ears go bare than wear something conservative, common or stingy in spirit. Voluptuous pearls, however, are always acceptable.

Bombshells are innocently inappropriate with their office wear and have been known to wear fancy jewelry to international conferences. Marilyn Monroe in *As Young As You Feel* wears a fitted white dress held at the shoulders with large diamond buttons, far more suited for evening wear. A Bombshell is not going to water down her style just because she's going to her day job.

Bombshells occasionally wear sapphires, usually accompanied by diamonds and pearls. They have also been known to wear coral or turquoise while vacationing in balmy climates.

Bombshells are known to sell their jewelry for worthy causes[1] and will sell diamonds to help friends and lovers.[2]

Some Bombshells count on their own sparkle. Of diamonds, Kim Novak said, "I think they're rather foolish. How can a woman feel that she can compete with them. You wouldn't purposely stand next to the most beautiful woman in the room."

THE ESSENTIAL BOMBSHELL JEWELRY WARDROBE

Two pairs (minimum) dangling diamond or
rhinestone earrings

Dangling faux pearl earrings

Large diamond or rhinestone brooch

One diamond or rhinestone bracelet

Large diamond or rhinestone necklace;
sapphire optional

One silver ankle bracelet (never under nylons)

Two or more pairs of large hoop earrings in silver
or platinum or gold

Charm bracelet

---

1 Brigitte Bardot sold 116 items at auction in Paris, including an 8.36-carat diamond that her husband Gunther Sachs gave her a decade after their divorce and a diamond Cartier bracelet, and raised $500,000 for her animal protection agency.

2 Elizabeth Taylor sold a 69.42-carat ring from Richard Burton to raise money for politician flame John Warner.

Bombshell
Underpinnings

A Bombshell is just as concerned with what isn't seen as what is. She doesn't care if a man is going to see her stockings or garter belt, and there is a good chance that he will as she's getting out of a cab or standing over a grating. This is her inner ammunition. While the Bombshell is not given to gauche displays or exhibitionism per se, in the spirit of the moment she might bend over a little too far, let the breeze do its thing or reveal a lot more than a little leg. Bombshells cause scandals all the time.[1] They don't plan to, it just happens.

Sophia Loren flashes her red-panty–clad derrière while dancing in *The Pride and the Passion*. Marilyn Monroe cheerfully showed all in the famous white-dress-blowing-up *Seven Year Itch* publicity photo taken on Lexington Avenue.

---

1 One Italian magazine cover featured Sophia Loren lifting her skirts so high that Italian police confiscated the entire issue and fined the publishers for an "offense against public decency."

Bras

When it comes to bras it's all or nothing. Bras with titles go over big with the Bombshell. The "Famous 502" by Exquisite Form is her favorite sweater bra. Its crescent understitching creates an alert, pointed effect. When the Bombshell goes for architecture, she wants suspension. Jane Russell had it in *The Outlaw*. Howard Hughes designed her bra, the "cantilever," using bridge technology. Never mind that she's wearing peasant clothes.

Contrary to popular opinion, the Bombshell does not shop at Frederick's of Hollywood unless it's an emergency or for the Cadillac, her favorite bra for over-the-top cleavage. She adores decorative trims and/or contrasting lace and has a weakness for combinations like black and champagne. The Bombshell will own several merry widows by Lady Marlene and Warner in black, white, or black with an underlay of pink or champagne. She also has underwire demi-bras by La Perla and Chantelle in mesh, lace, eyelet and silk for the ultimate décolletage. The Bombshell never wears bras in wild colors. She saves that for panties.

Bombshells are also famous for bralessness. A little bounce, a little jiggle, the Bombshell is never apologetic for being a woman. Brigitte Bardot frequently went without a bra, Jean Harlow wore slinky satin gowns with nothing underneath, and Kim Novak had no use for them. Hollywood tried to make her over, but the one thing she wouldn't dispense with was not wearing a brassiere. When she filmed *Picnic* she was told that a girl in the Midwest would always wear a bra. "Well," she said, "I was brought up in the Midwest, and I never wore a bra."

Kim Novak claimed to shun girdles, as well. She once said, "I like my comfort. If you have nothing to hide, why hide it?" Marilyn Monroe sang "Happy Birthday" to the president in public without underpinnings in a virtually see-through gown.

Panties

There is only one rule: Panty lines are unacceptable. Bombshells like panties in white, lavender, pale pink, hot pink, champagne, yellow, black, red, turquoise, zebra, leopard and polka dots. Underpants may be sheer, ruffled, lace, silk, eyelet or plain cotton in boy-cut, string bikini or classic briefs. Whenever possible, the Bombshell prefers panties of French, Swiss or Italian origin, but she has the imagination to find the perfect little number at JCPenney. The Bombshell finds thongs uncomfortable and would rather wear nothing at all.[2] She consults her full-length mirror after getting dressed and if her underpants show, off they come.

The Garter Belt

The Bombshell respects tradition. Corsetier Rigby & Peller was founded in 1939 and in 1956 was granted the Royal Warrant as corsetier to HM Queen Elizabeth II and soon after to HM the Queen Mother. This makes the Rigby & Peller garter belts the first choice of the Bombshell. She has them in black, champagne and ivory lace. She also has several other brands in cotton, in white, pink, yellow or baby blue. These will be from JCPenney.

Stockings

Unless it's dance class, in which case the Bombshell will wear tights—Capezio and Freed of London—pantyhose are not Bombshell material. They're too efficient, confining, pedestrian and lacking in intrigue. It's no stockings and a naked leg or a garter belt and stockings. These may be silk or nylon, seamed or not. Climate has nothing to do with the Bombshell's decision to wear stockings or go without. Jane Russell wears them on a balmy South Seas cruise in the film *Macao.* But Bombshells in the middle of winter have been known to go bare-legged for the sake of their bare-toed san-

---

2 Earl Wilson in *Show Business Laid Bare* writes, "Once at a night party at Toots Shor's restaurant, Marilyn, not wearing any pants that night, sat down on a chair and got splinters in her famous posterior. The splinters went through her thin dress. My wife took Marilyn to the powder room and extracted the splinters."

dals or peekaboo pumps. In the film . . . *And God Created Woman*, Brigitte Bardot forsakes all hosiery and goes barefoot at every opportunity.

Where the Bombshell Shops for Underpinnings

The Bombshell prefers boutiques for her lingerie, preferably with sleek rococo or Empire period furniture, not mass chains or anything found in a mall.

La Perla in New York
La Petite Coquette in New York
Only Hearts in Los Angeles

Bombshells in the Buff

You never know when a Bombshell might bare all. In *Pandora and the Flying Dutchman*, Ava Gardner strips off ballgown, cape and stockings, leaving her fiancé ashore, and swims naked to a schooner anchored in the bay to introduce herself to the owner played by James Mason. In *The Cabin in the Cotton*, a lithe, blonde Bette Davis slips into her walk-in closet, leaving the door ajar with her fiancé in the room and says, "Turn your back while I get into something more restful." To a Bombshell, that's her birthday suit.

Almost every Bombshell starts out posing naked for something or other. A calendar, a magazine, a so-called photographer. Sometimes she poses nude after she is famous.

The Bombshell loves to take her clothes off. In *Come Dance with Me!*, Brigitte Bardot declares, "When I'm naked I lose all my complexes." Marilyn Monroe liked to give telephone interviews in the nude. Once she gave one in front of the publicist Joe Wohlander. "I'm only comfortable when I'm naked," she said.

According to Earl Wilson in his book *Show Business Laid Bare,* Marilyn Monroe "was always demanding more and more nudity which she knew was good for her. When she was filming *The Seven Year Itch* with Tom Ewell in 1954 . . . she wanted to do a nude love scene, which in those years was unthinkable."

In 1983, Kim Basinger posed nude for eight pages of *Playboy.* "It's my ballgame," she told the *Daily News* in 1987. "We shoot the pictures, I choose the pictures, and then we're going to approach sixteen guys in the industry—Fellini, Bob Fosse—and show them the pictures, and say, 'What do you think?' And then I'm going to have lunch with them. I just meant it to be, 'Hey, hey, I'm here.' But everybody—my agents, my publicists, my lawyers—said, 'It'll ruin you.' I said, 'Fine, let it ruin me.' I needed—I don't mean this as a pun—exposure."

Gina Lollobrigida disdained such practices. "I would never pose for one of those bunny magazines," she told the *New York Sunday News* in 1971. "No, never. I don't need this kind of picture. I'm sexy fully dressed," she said. Her outfit that day: a netted see-through dress.

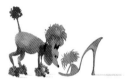

BOMBSHELL SLEEP & LOUNGEWEAR

A Bombshell knows that anything can happen in the middle of the night—a fire, an earthquake, a party—and dresses for the occasion. Filmy is the operative word. A Bombshell does not necessarily sleep in her sleepwear, but may lounge in it and drape it across her folding screen or a chair before going to bed. "I adore to have a lot of nightdresses," Brigitte Bardot said. "But in my closet, not on me."

The Bombshell, when asked what she sleeps in, has been known to say, "Chanel No. 5."

A Bombshell understands protocol and under no circumstances wears sleepwear or intimate apparel in public, except in case of abovementioned emergencies. She will, for example, allow herself to be photographed in a sheer negligée if posing in her bed, on the stairs to the bedroom, or even by the door, as long as it's inside.

The Bombshell's sleepwear collection includes a full-length negligée of cream lace with or without rhinestones, a lace negligée, sheer baby doll pajamas in pink, black and champagne, a satin charmeuse gown with matching peignoir, a well-fitted white slip, a well-fitted black slip, Chinese pajamas in jade with a gold pattern, a kimono in sky blue silk, various diaphanous bed jackets, several knee-length sheer nightgowns (black or champagne only), and two nightshirts, one in red silk and one in fine cotton embroidered with her initials.

Inspired by the drapery of ancient Greek statues—think caryatids on the Acropolis—the Bombshell considers the bed sheet to be an impromptu part of the boudoir wardrobe, your bedroom or hers. She considers the sheet appropriately demure for answering room service, standing on balconies, hanging out of windows, seeing lovers to the door, posing for photographs and signing for UPS packages. Her sheet preference is white, cotton only, with a high thread count. Bombshells are too sensitive to sleep on polyester.

Towels are also considered to be appropriate cover.

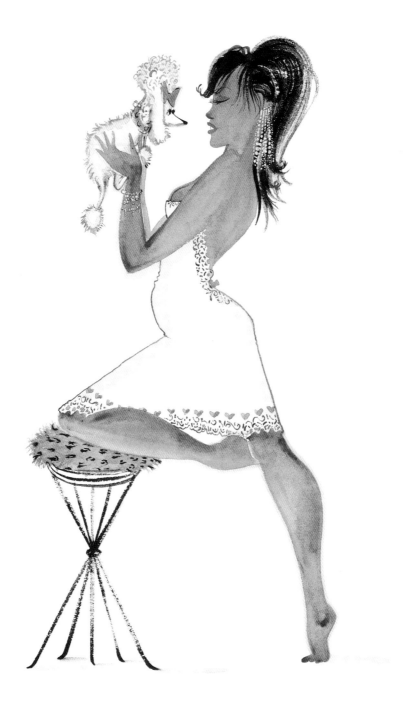

BOMBSHELL PERFUME

She makes a great entrance. Crosses her legs seductively, curls, stretches or perches on divans, sofas, bar stools. But it is her perfume that finally puts you in her thrall. A Bombshell does not choose her scent cavalierly. She has read the famous line by the early twentieth-century French poet Paul Valéry, "There is no future for a woman who does not use perfume properly," and taken it to heart. A Bombshell knows the Bombshell fragrances. She has tried them all and knows which ones heighten her body chemistry and mood. She might love Chanel No. 5 on a tester strip, its romantic inclinations, its provenance, its seductive, electric French aura, but if it argues with her own essence, she'll keep looking.

With rare exception, Bombshells wear classic, full-flowered, even old-fashioned perfumes but never anything skinny, streamlined, vulgar or loud. In short, nothing beneath her, or that will upstage.

The less clothing a Bombshell wears, the more perfume she dons. Perfumes, in fact, may be described with the same terms as Bombshells: *Irresistible. Seductive. Voluptuous.*

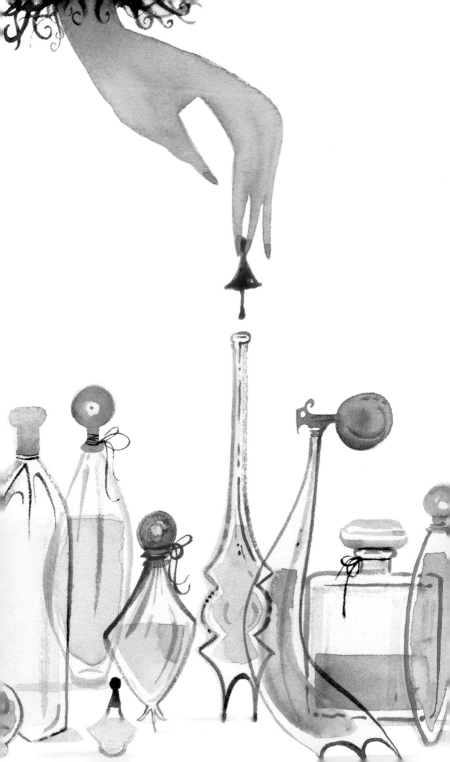

Full-bodied. A Bombshell always calls her scent *perfume*, never *fragrance*, even if it's eau de toilette.

Arpège by Lanvin

Fragile and sumptuous simultaneously, Arpège is a complicated fragrance with a heart of rose, coriander, mimosa, jasmine and geranium. It is the kind of perfume that quietly envelops—terribly suggestive and erotic without ever being obvious. Simply put, Arpège is lazily provocative and has been disarming anyone within olfactory range since 1927. Sit next to a Bombshell wearing Arpège and you'll eventually wonder, *What hit me?* Best in old-world surroundings, Scottish castles, Russian tea rooms or any place with crystal chandeliers, Arpège adores low-cut dresses, but doesn't rely on them. Arpège appreciates diamonds but is really better suited for less obvious stones—Russian amber, vintage tiger's eye, garnets, carnelian; think estate jewelry.

Arpège is not recommended for the young and inexperienced Bombshell. Seasoned Bombshells know that this fragrance, like a fine wine, needs a little time to warm up. (Celebrity user: Jayne Mansfield in *Will Success Spoil Rock Hunter?*)

Chanel

The Bombshell wears them all: No. 5, No. 19, No. 22, Coco, Cristalle, except for Allure, which she might buy for a niece, but finds too girlish for herself.

No. 19: shimmering and mysterious, No. 19 is best suited for Bombshells with introspective tendencies. At first sniff it's rather meadowlike and green—galbanum, hyacinth, neroli and bergamot compose the top notes, but its heart, like the Bombshell's, is romantic and complex, with deep, woodsy notes of the enchanted forest variety.

No. 22 is a highly floral scent best suited to highly cheerful Bombshells. Said to "shimmer like champagne bubbles" it virtually sings (with a soft, elegant tremor) with a top note of orange blossom and bergamot and has an exotic floral heart that includes deliriously happy tuberose. A Bombshell might wear this fragrance on a first date, as it will let her own personality steal the limelight. Timeless. Ageless. Seasonless. (Celebrity user: Catherine Deneuve)

Coco is made for brunette Bombshells with big personalities. The ingredients, of course, are exotic—Comoros Islands orange blossom, Spice Islands clove bud, Caribbean cascarilla, Bulgarian rose, Indian jasmine, Mysore sandalwood—nothing shy here. Think flamboyance, low-cut red dresses, the assertive seductive power of Jane Russell in *Macao*. It's what Bombshells wear to tango class; too distracting for the office.

Cristalle: exciting, electric, green and alert, a Bombshell splashes on Cristalle when she doesn't have time for coffee and simply smells her wrist when she needs a pick-me-up. It elevates her spirits without making her jittery.

Diorissimo by Christian Dior

A Bombshell wouldn't dream of exercising without the appropriate fragrance. It must be light, clean, rapturous and give her a sense of hope. Inspired by the delicate, quivering lily of the valley, Diorissimo is her favorite. It makes her feel ethereal, almost weightless and always optimistic. Diorissimo is the Bombshell choice for tennis, hiking, working out with weights and badminton.

Femme by Rochas

A feminine, warm, embracing, sweater-girl scent. Perfect for intimate affairs in small rooms, in front of fireplaces, French restaurants. Ideal for evening tweeds; snug cashmere twinsets in taupe, ivory, peach and black; dark, clingy knits and cocktail dresses. Femme adores plunging necklines which are best with an understated perfume that's a little woodsy, soft and complex. (Celebrity user: Mae West)

Fracas by Piguet

Introduced in 1945 by Paris couturier Robert Piguet. Black-glove elegant and as exuberant as a blown kiss, Fracas is the ultimate cocktail fragrance. With its outstanding top note of tuberose, Fracas is like an exclamation point of hot pink. (Flamingo pink lip color completes the sensation.) It's appropriate for all seasons and is most stunning with black in crepe, velvet, brocade, silk and cashmere. Potent and romantic enough to scent serious love letters. (Celebrity user: Kim Basinger)

Gardenia Passion by Annick Goutal

Intense. Dramatic. Think laughter, the kind where your head is thrown back in abandon. The Bombshell adores it on summer nights in outdoor cafes, lawn and gazebo parties. Enhanced by white, off white, oyster and ivory silk satin, eyelet and chiffon.

Jicky by Guerlain

At first sniff, Jicky appears too complex, introverted and shy for a Bombshell. Created at the end of the nineteenth century, it is a perfume of great intelligence and refinement, with a pointed top note of citrus/bergamot and a sweet, balsamic heart of jasmine, rose and sultry orris. Its base, however, purrs with exotic animal undercurrents of civet and leather. Jicky is marvelous, in fact, with just about anything a Bombshell is likely to lounge in from ivory charmeuse nightgowns and pale pink baby dolls to red Chinese silk pajamas. It is the kind of perfume that luxuriously scents lingerie, too, but it also likes to spend time out of the house. French Bombshells understand the power of understatement. Colette, one of the Bombshell's favorite French writers, is said to have worn it. (Celebrity user: Brigitte Bardot)

Joy by Jean Patou

Voluptuous, full-flowered Joy is a favorite of the Bombshell, though she would never buy it for herself. As Joy is the costliest perfume in the world, she expects to receive it as a gift. Bombshells of great charm have been known to have so many bottles of Joy at one time that they become positively reckless, dabbing it on letters, scenting lingerie, splashing it into the bath, scenting their poodles. Created for the French couturier Jean Patou, who wanted a fragrance that would be "free from vulgarity . . . impudent, crazy and extravagant beyond reason," Joy has dominant notes of jasmine and rose mingled with more than one hundred essences. The Bombshell loves Joy with low-cut dresses and lots of rocks. (Celebrity users: Josephine Baker, Gloria Swanson and Marilyn Monroe)

L'Heure Bleue by Guerlain

A summer evening scent that spans a poetic range of romantic emotions, this is the fragrance to wear when falling in love. Eternally fresh, woodsy, powdery and feminine with a spicy heart of clove, it adores filmy, gauzy, velvety blue, violet and periwinkle anything. Jacques Guerlain is said to have been moved by the twilight hour when the sky has lost its sun but has not yet found its stars. Young Bombshells play dress-up in this charming, seductive scent. L'Heure Bleue gives the fully blossomed Bombshell an aura as luminous as pearls. (Celebrity user: Patricia Arquette)

Mitsouko by Guerlain

Caution. This rich fragrance with a mandarin/peach top note is only to be worn under the cover of night. Mitsouko has more sensuous layers to unpeel than Rita Hayworth dancing the Dance of the Seven Veils as Salome. Mitsouko means mystery in Japanese, and this perfume, with deep notes of cinnamon, clove and myrrh, promises to reveal a voluptuous secret before daybreak. A favorite of the original Bombshell, Jean Harlow (famous for shunning underlayers), Mitsouko unfolds like a fragrant flower that opens only at night. (Celebrity user: Jean Harlow)

My Sin by Lanvin

Unleash the forbidden, intoxicating radiance of Pandora's box and you've experienced My Sin. This is perhaps the most amazing fragrance ever created. My Sin opens doors to the subconscious: it is an explosion of innocence and sensuality. My Sin is heady; the quintessential Bombshell fragrance. It is more wild than wild, reckless, curved, high-throttle, empowered with dreams. Its top note of fast-lane aldehydes and Versailles-garden citrus awakens primordial passions; vanilla, vetiver, sandalwood and civet give it depth. It is the fragrance of Venus; the ultimate perfume of the goddess.

My Sin is alarming and sexually provocative at first but settles into filmy desire. Jam packed with emotion, My Sin sparkles across the room and smolders upon intimacy. A vintage bottle turns up now and then, but this beautiful, shimmering, coy perfume is no longer made. How it came to be extinct is a mystery. It lived fast, faded too soon. (Celebrity user: Jayne Mansfield in *Promises! Promises!*)

Norell by Revlon

An elegant, luxurious, white-gloved floral scent with a hyacinth top note, Norell is what the Bombshell wears when mingling at political fund-raisers in the late summer. At least it certainly seems polite at first. All American, very polished, cool and glamorous but with something a little dangerous simmering underneath. Think Elizabeth Taylor in *A Place in the Sun*. Good with eyelet, charmeuse, strapless white gowns. (Celebrity user: Faye Dunaway)

Nude by Bill Blass

First, the name. It's irresistible to the Bombshell. It makes her think of slipping out of her bathing suit on a deserted beach. Often a Bombshell will wear this fragrance when there's a good chance she will be undressed by someone. A striking floral composition, Nude is actually more gauzy and filmy than naked in its evocation, and creates a mental state of near undress.

Shalimar by Guerlain

The Bombshell adores the Shalimar story. She falls for it every time. Sanskrit for "abode of love," Shalimar is named for the lush gardens of the Taj Mahal, created by an Indian emperor for his queen. Shamelessly feminine, outrageously romantic, Shalimar has a heart of jasmine, rose, heliotrope and iris. (Celebrity users: Gina Lollobrigida and Rita Hayworth)

Spring Flower by Creed

That pink bottle is why she smelled it in the first place, but she was head over heels once it blossomed on her pulse points. The Bombshell wouldn't dream of attending a smelly sporting event without the appropriate fragrance, and Spring Flower is one of her high-pitched floral favorites. She relies

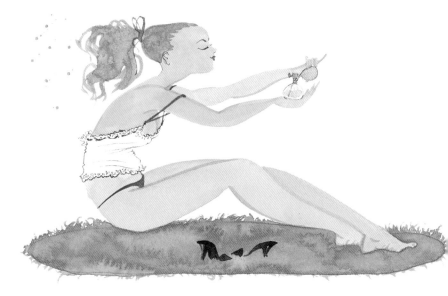

on it for the Triple Crown, heavyweight championships and polo matches.

Tabu by Dana

This is not a scent for the faint-hearted Bombshell. Potent and spicy with a "narcotic" floral heart, this scent is the velvety, sizzling starter for many a Bombshell and is most fitting for those with an uninhibited nature. Tabu comes on as strong and sexy as Dorothy Dandridge playing the free-spirited *Carmen Jones*, Gina Lollobrigida in *Trapeze*, Ava Gardner in *The Barefoot Contessa*. Remarkably versatile, it goes with wine-colored velvet, black velvet and all manner of wild peasant garb.

Tabac Blond by Caron

Created in 1919 when perfume became emancipated from its strictly feminine bouquets (the same year Gloria Swanson introduced the nude bathing scene in the film *Male and Female*), Tabac Blond is one of the earthiest, most exciting and sensual of the Bombshell fragrances. Unfazed by time, shockingly modern, Tabac Blond reminds the Bombshell of her first date with a guy with wheels. That is to say, it has lover's lane nostalgia as well as elegance going for it. It is a youthful scent, combining lusty leather and tobacco notes with innocent, sing-songy, powdery carnation, iris and ylang-ylang and is recommended for Bombshells with wanderlust. Hair color? Not an issue. Necklines? Collarbones at the very least should show. Comfortable in fast cars, slow cars, grand cafes in Vienna, casinos in Monte Carlo, nightclubs any-where. Strangely, Tabac Blond is perfect for a romantic autumn weekend and dramatic enough for the opera. (Too naughty for high tea.) If you must travel light and Tabac Blond suits you, this is the perfume to grab. It was difficult to find in the United States until recently when the Caron shop opened on Madison Avenue. Bombshells love its exclusivity.

Other Bombshell Perfumes from Caron

Narcisse Noir. An exotic, voluptuous, daring, sensual scent immortalized by Gloria Swanson in *Sunset Boulevard.*

Narcisse Blanc. A very feminine scent with delicate notes of neroli, orange blossom and jasmine that's not so innocent once it warms up.

Nuit de Noel. Imagine seeing Paris on a snowy, wintry night from the top of the Eiffel Tower while sipping champagne. Created in 1922, this warming, heartful scent pays homage to the roaring twenties with an effect so uplifting it's dizzying.

Vent Vert by Balmain

It tries to be breezy and green, but Vent Vert is not quite as innocent as it appears at first whiff. How could it be with a base of oak moss, sandalwood, sage, iris, amber and musk? Still it evokes summer. Think gingham dresses (fitted), white piqué and off-the-shoulder peasant blouses with Capri pants, a head scarf and jeweled sandals. (Celebrity user: Brigitte Bardot)

White Shoulders
by Evyan

Someone the Bombshell admired in her youth wore this delicate, whispering perfume with a slightly risqué base note—a baby-sitter, a teacher, the aunt with the coral lipstick and all the wigs, the one who sang gospel and told her about writing thank-you letters (see Stationery, page 117). To the Bombshell it's the most polite fragrance there is, the kind she wears to church.

Youth Dew by Estée Lauder

It takes a certain type of Bombshell to get away with the spicy *wow* of Youth Dew. Svelte and subtle it's not. Youth Dew parades around practically naked, hitting you over the head with all its voluptuous curves. Yet it's also very old-fashioned and flaunts its powdery notes. It's as warming as cognac (legend has it that Youth Dew was based on a formula created for a Russian princess; she must have been the uninhibited sort), but somehow evokes a thick, sultry southern atmosphere mingled with dusting powder and the sexy aroma of fruit that's almost a little too ripe. Think of an ivory stiletto slipping off an arched foot on a hot day and the powdery scent emanating from chiffoned cleavage (nothing underneath) where ropes of coral and pearls tangle. The Bombshell in question, even if she's reading a gentle passage from Keats from her white porch swing, will be sipping something much stronger than champagne. (Celebrity users: Dolores Del Rio, Gloria Swanson, Joan Crawford)

Perfumes a Bombshell Never Wears

Anything that smells like food: vanilla; single-fruit notes like strawberry or apple. Jolting, loud or overwhelming fragrances like Opium, Poison and Giorgio. Overtly green scents like Calyx. Laura Ashley—too innocent. Obsession. CK One. Lauren. Eternity. Musk. Patchouli. Tea Rose. Charlie.

Scents Bombshells Like on Men

When it comes to men's colognes, the Bombshell has definite ideas. She trusts anything worn by Cary Grant, Gary Cooper, Frank Sinatra, Errol Flynn, Douglas Fairbanks and her dad. She will also have a nostalgic attachment to anything worn by her first boyfriend.

The Bombshell appreciates old-fashioned classics like Old Spice, which smells handsome, masculine, reliable and trustworthy, and the more daredevil manly fifties classic, Aqua Velva Ice Blue.

In addition, she likes fragrances she can borrow. These include: Christian Dior's Eau Sauvage, Guerlain's Habit Rouge and Equipage by Hermès, Acqua di Parma (Ava Gardner adored it) and Vetivert, preferably from a small shop in New Orleans called Hové that the Bombshell visited during Mardi Gras one year.

MASCULINE NOTES

Cary Grant:
Acqua di Parma

Guerlain's Eau Impériale
Creed's Green Irish Tweed

Gary Cooper:
Creed's Epicea

Frank Sinatra:
Creed's Bois du Portugal

Errol Flynn:
Creed's Bois de Cedrat

Douglas Fairbanks:
Creed's Citrus Bigarrade
(Originally created for the Duke and
Duchess of Windsor.)

Where Bombshells Buy Perfume

Aedes de Venustas, Christopher Street, New York
(Leopard prints, wall-to-wall carpeting, baroque
furniture, personal attention, a cute little dog.)

Saks Fifth Avenue

Boyd's, Madison Avenue, New York

Caron, Madison Avenue, New York

Annick Goutal, Paris, France

Guerlain, Paris, France

Chanel, Rodeo Drive, Los Angeles

Bombshell Handbags

The Bombshell likes a good fit. She chooses a handbag the way she chooses a slip—it's not just about looks. It should feel snug, well-proportioned, natural, a part of her. The Bombshell likes classic styles in small to medium sizes. Messenger bags, backpacks and briefcases are out of the question—too utilitarian. Never trendy or flamboyant, the Bombshell handbag is not meant to draw attention or distract, but rather to complement.

The Top Handle Bag

The Bombshell refers to this as her pocketbook. Always her first choice for day, she likes a ladylike bag in a color and fabric that goes with her shoes. Deceptively prim and proper, the top handle bag allows her to keep her shoulders thrown back and accentuate her sashay. Simple, square shapes are popular with the Bombshell. No flashy hardware, overt logos or unreasonable embellishments. She will have these in straw with tortoiseshell trim, leather in white, black, navy, oxblood, red or taupe and an animal print or two. The Bombshell can't bear a beat-up handbag. She goes for a good patina on her leather, but when it shows too much wear and tear, she gives it to that little girl down the hall.

The Day or Envelope Clutch

This is the clutch that swings in her hand or goes under the arm. The one she'll bring if there's a chance she may end up at a cocktail party that evening. They are sleek, but substantial enough to hold a paperback. She likes these in all fabrics and colors from black macramé to silk to leather.

The Shoulder Bag

This is not the Bombshell's first choice. Since she never has owned or will own an attaché or tote, this is the bag she will use to carry memoirs, scripts, head shots, contracts, etc. It will be at least 8½ by 11 inches with a very short strap to allow a narrow range of motion.

Bombshell Day Bags

Chanel (never quilted)
Christian Dior
Fendi
Ferragamo
Gucci
Hermès Kelly Bag
Lambertson/Truex
Lana Marks
Prada
Mark Cross, vintage

What's in Her Day Bag

Chiclets or Juicy Fruit

Comb

Compact (loose powder in case)

Needle and thread from a hotel (she'll never use it)

Curious George notebook or a memo pad
from Asprey & Garrard

Tiny tin of aspirin

Lipstick

Napkin from the Plaza bathroom

Slim Tiffany blue ballpoint pen

Ink marks from Tiffany pen

Postcard stamps

Lucky silver dollar

Tiny perfume atomizer

Cocktail umbrella

Wayward stones from jewelry she means to have repaired

Pink eraser

Fortune cookies

Assorted coat check stubs

A tattered roll of butter rum LifeSavers

There is no Filofax or electronic calendar; the
Bombshell has faith in her inner clock and prefers to memo-
rize her schedule or scribble appointment times, etc., on
small pieces of paper.

The Bombshell does not own a cell phone but she'll
gladly borrow yours.

The Evening Clutch

This is where she gets fancy. Usually rectangular, no longer than asparagus, as long as it's glamorous just about anything goes—black velvet, silk shantung, Chinese prints in red or champagne, Indian embroidery with metallic threads, passementerie, beading, paillettes. Never a minaudière encrusted with stones or anything in the shape of animal, vegetable or mineral. The Bombshell's evening bag will inevitably be ivory, white, black, pale pink or a color chosen to match her gown. The inside of the evening clutch is just as important to the Bombshell—she likes them silk-lined—and she adores the kind that comes with a little mirror. The Bombshell loves a rhinestone or pearl clasp, but not one so large that it competes with her jewelry.

Bombshell Evening Bags

Anya Hindmarch
Something silk from Chinatown
Handmade bag by Leo Miller in Paris

What's in Her Evening Clutch

Lipstick, compact, handkerchief, keys and enough change for a phone call.

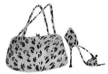

Bombshell Scarves

Unless reading Hemingway on a beach in Key West (large-brimmed straw hat, the bigger the better), a hat is never welcome. But no Bombshell can resist a scarf. Oversized, tiny, sheer, beaded, scalloped—she works them all. But one thing's for sure, she never covers her chest. Never. A Bombshell picks up scarves in airports, on road trips or whenever she needs a little cheering up. Needless to say, she has quite a collection. The Bombshell never hand-launders her scarves, but has them dry cleaned or presses them between the dictionary and world atlas.

The Oblongs

The Bombshell has these in two sizes: 42 by 11 inches and 64 by 19 inches. She wears the smaller one as a headband knotted behind one ear so it drapes over her shoulder the way Elizabeth Taylor wears hers at the beach in *Suddenly, Last Summer*. The Bombshell wears the oblong in this fashion after the beach, on the boardwalk and to outdoor cafes in Cannes, St. Tropez, etc. She likes these in breezy chiffons and in whatever color matches her bathing suit. She also likes polka dots. The Bombshell wears the larger oblong tossed around the neck so it floats down her back like wings. On extremely windy days she will wrap it once around her neck. The Bombshell likes this look with strapless, backless and halter tops. She also wears it with tight cashmere roundneck sweaters to create a little movement. The large oblong is also considered an evening wrap and she will have gloves to match. It will be in white, black, sequined black, lavender chiffon or polka dots. For evening convertible driving, the Bombshell may wear the oblong in white chiffon far back over the head and wrapped to trail down her back (see Elizabeth Taylor in *A Place in the Sun*).

The Squares

THE SMALL SQUARE OR BANDANNA OR KERCHIEF

This scarf will be no larger than 19 inches. The Bombshell wears it tied behind her head primarily in Montana and the other cowboy states. She wears the kerchief on horseback, in trucks, Jeeps, on hay rides and when roasting marshmallows. It will be in cotton in any color that pleases her except for black, which she considers unsuitable for the great outdoors. The Bombshell will also have a kerchief in white eyelet, a traditional bandanna print or the print or color that matches her bikini. The Bombshell will also wear the cotton kerchief knotted around the neck with sporty attire like dungarees.

The Traditional Square

This scarf measures 30 inches square. It is worn on the head, wrapped around the neck and tied in back. The Bombshell considers this her casual driving scarf and prefers to wear it when the top is down. This scarf is expressly worn with sunglasses. The Bombshell likes these squares in heavy silk with hand-rolled edges in white, taupe, ivory, hot pink, champagne and polka dots. Hermès, Pucci, Echo and Vera are the Bombshell's favorites. In a pinch, the traditional square may be folded into a triangle and tied in the back to be worn as a top.

The Oversized Square or Sarong

This will be at least 49 inches square and may be batik, exotic floral or sheer gauze. While the Bombshell might wrap an oversized square around her shoulders she feels more inclined to knot it around her hips sarong-style. Dorothy Lamour made her sarong debut in *The Road to Singapore* in 1940 and Bombshells have been following suit ever since. Having spent so much time running around the house and posing in towels, it was only a matter of time before she went public with this look. A Bombshell will have two to ten sarong-style squares in her drawer, at least one with fringe. Several match bikini tops.

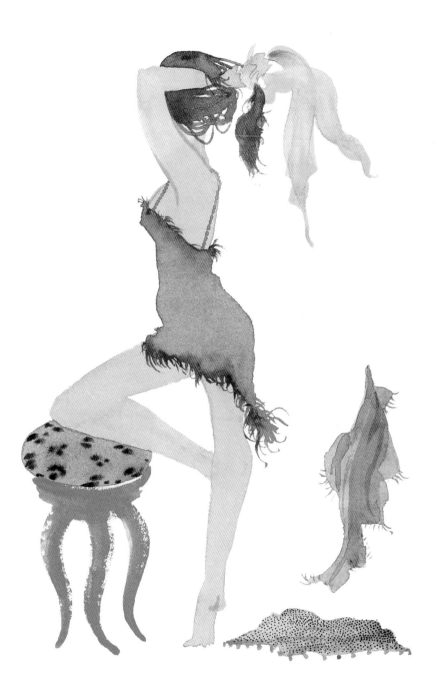

Bombshell Footwear
(or At Her Feet)

Bombshell footwear always looks like it's about to be kicked off or as if it's been hastily slipped on after getting out of the tub.

Any peekaboo sandal will be the first choice of a Bombshell, even in the coldest of weather. The Bombshell favors an open toe—she does this, confident people will take care that she is warm. Doors are opened for her and cars are sent for her. Her escort, the concierge and bystanders leap at the opportunity to rub her feet at the slightest sign of a chill. (The Bombshell prefers bare legs, of course, to stockings of any kind, despite the cold.) The look and effect she accomplishes with open toes and sandals is worth the discomfort.

Mules

The mule is a complicated shoe for the Bombshell. It would appear to be the ideal shoe, but is actually somewhat complex because of the fine line the Bombshell eternally walks. A Bombshell is not trashy, trampy or vampy. Under no circumstances does she wear lingerie in public, and the mule, if recklessly chosen, can resemble a bedroom accessory. A Bombshell, therefore, will absolutely wear the appropriate mule with lingerie, over breakfast and before bed. At-home mules are rather tall; the width of the heel, however, is purely personal to the specific Bombshell and the accompanying lingerie, which will, of course, match. It's safe to say that these are in black, baby blue, pink, champagne or white

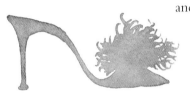 and are made of fluff, feathers or satin. She considers her feet to be one of her most stunning features and would never hide them with anything garish or wildly printed. Think Jayne Mansfield in *Will Success Spoil Rock Hunter?*

For public wear, the Bombshell chooses a simple mule—never spike-heeled or platformed and no front strap thicker than your average Hershey's chocolate bar. White glove elegance is de rigueur. No feathers, no sequins, no appliqués, no lamé. Leather, patent leather, possibly suede, Lucite of course, and taffeta for evening are acceptable fabrics for public mule wearing.

Slingbacks

The strap must be string thin—virtually invisible, an optical illusion. No buckles or clasps larger than a small housefly. We see her bare heel, but only the slightest glimpse of the strap itself—hardly substantial enough to be holding her shoe snugly to her foot. This is one of the Bombshell's favorite gravity-defying acts.

She likes these shoes in neutral fleshy tones—beige, cream, cafe, ivory, clear or white to create a long, uninterrupted line from leg to foot—the leg that goes on forever à la *The Seven Year Itch*. However, a teeny, tiny black strap done as delicately as lingerie works nicely on a Bombshell. Think Fellini films, circa 1950.

The Pump

The pump is not the first choice of the Bombshell. Unless it shows toe cleavage and has a high heel, or is see-through like the ones Brigitte Bardot wears in *Contempt*, the pump is too demure and/or businesslike for a Bombshell.

For day, she will consider a pump only if she's wearing a shapely suit. There can be minimal roundness to the toe—she prefers to make a point—and the heel should be at least four inches tall.

With a floor-length gown, the Bombshell prefers a cut-out toe. Operas, charity balls, and public appearances require that she be at her gravity-defying best. In these instances there is no limit to how high her heel can go.

Barefeet

Bombshells are famous for their barefootedness (think Bardot in . . . *And God Created Woman*, Ava Gardner in *The Barefoot Contessa,* Marilyn Monroe in *Some Like It Hot*, Kim Novak in *Bell, Book and Candle*).

Bombshells are often barefoot because they have nothing else on. But it is widely known that shoes are the first article of clothing they take off.

Marilyn Monroe in *The Misfits* dances barefoot with Eli Wallach and Clark Gable. In this movie she does two things that Bombshells always do: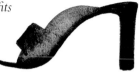

1 Kicks off her shoes.
2 Walks or stands on the balls of her feet as if she is still wearing high heels. The idea is that she is light as a feather. Elevated. High on life.

Bombshell Heels

Ferragamo, vintage
(Marilyn was definitely onto something.)

Manolo Blahnik

Dolce & Gabbana

Charles Jourdan

Jimmy Choo

Richard Tyler

Sigerson Morrison (sandals only)

Ernesto Esposito

Bernard Figueroa

Christian Louboutin (The look is understated and glamorous, the soles are shiny red and she likes having her feet, especially bare feet, next to his fancy signature.)

Casual Footwear

Keds sneakers

Straw slippers from Agnès b. or Chinatown

Beaded Minnetonka moccasins
(The originals. These are appropriate cabin
and ranch wear with dungarees.)

Freed of London ballet slippers
(The pink is peachy, like lingerie. She also has black.)

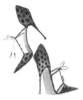

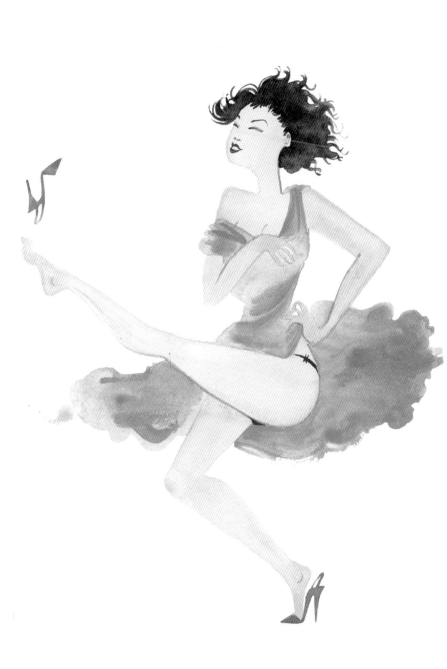

Bombshell Hair

First, there's the hairdresser. Every Bombshell has one. When Rita Hayworth left her husband Aly Khan, the note read, "Have flown with Thelma to Majorca. Will phone you from there. Love, Rita." Thelma was her hairdresser. The Bombshell travels with hairdresser in tow, otherwise she bonds with the first good one she meets. In *Promises! Promises!*, Jayne Mansfield instantly takes to Babbette, the cruise ship's hairdresser. When she announces she's pregnant, his idea of a baby shower gift is a collection of wigs.

The Bombshell lists her hairdresser in her address book under "In Case of Emergency, Contact . . . " This is not just because he or she understands roots, volume and lift, but rather because he or she listens. The hairdresser has seen her moods, heartbreaks, and disappointments and knows when to make the kind of subtle adjustment in color or shape that will change everything.

A Bombshell is not born with Bombshell hair. She creates a signature look. Her hairdresser is her accomplice, her Svengali. Never pixie, never blunt, no haircuts with amusing names like Dutch boy or bob, never oversized, Bombshell hair is all about curves. It's a physical manifestation of the Bombshell personality; a sort of organized chaos with a little bounce. Loose, voluptuous, fluid. All reined in with a little Aqua Net or whatever her hairdresser prescribes.

Problem hair is one of the reasons the Bombshell is often late. Hair washed and styled to an unhappy conclusion is rewashed and reset; hairdressers and beauty salons are called in to save the day or evening.[1]

When it comes to styling, there are two main looks. Done and undone. Veronica Lake perfected the done variety with her famous peekaboo bang, a swell of tamed curves that coyly threatened to cover one eye. Long, blonde and parted at the side, the peekaboo bang was so emulated that the War Department issued a warning to women working in factories during World War II about the hazard of getting it caught in machinery. Being patriotic, another Bombshell quality, Lake chopped hers off.

Brigitte Bardot, on the other hand, excelled at bedroom hair. Long, slightly layered and almost always disheveled, her rumpled look was a calculated achievement.[2] "It's part of my personality," Bardot once declared, "undisciplined, like me."

The Bombshell doesn't run around changing her hair color. Once she's settled on a hue, that's it. Brigitte Bardot, a light-haired brunette by nature, might play around with dark

1 Hollywood gossip columnist Sid Skolsky wrote that Lana Turner insisted on washing her own hair, then frantically called her hairdresser to fix it when she couldn't "do a thing with it."

2 "You can't imagine," sighed Bardot's hairdresser, Jean-Pierre Berroyer (with whom she traveled). He revealed that the secret was very little water, dry shampoos every two days, lots of brushing, the least teasing possible and "shearing one centimeter every two weeks."

wigs in *Contempt*, but she never goes all the way. A Bombshell doesn't ditch her identity. She wouldn't change hair color for a movie role any more than she'd gain thirty pounds for a part. Exceptions to the hair-color rule usually prove disastrous. Even when everyone was declaring that blondes had more fun, Elizabeth Taylor didn't flirt with it. Roots, however, are a personal issue. Brigitte Bardot revealed hers shamelessly. But Marilyn Monroe kept hers private: she had them touched up every five days and carried hair whitener in her makeup case.

The Blonde Bombshell

Jean Harlow started the whole thing. With her ethereal halo of platinum hair, she became the archetypal love goddess. She put the blonde Bombshell on the map in the 1933 movie *Bombshell*. "The fans don't want to see the It Girl surrounded by an aura of motherhood," her publicist in the movie decreed. "I dubbed you the Hollywood Bombshell: Men. Scrapes. Dazzling clothes. A gorgeous pinwheel personality." The hair color of fairy tale heroines and victims, blonde is unthreatening, sexually open, childlike. It commands more attention than any other hair color and needs somebody who knows how to turn it on. Be prepared. Going blonde is letting the genie escape from the bottle.

The Brunette Bombshell

It's no coincidence Elizabeth Taylor was cast as Katharina in *The Taming of the Shrew*. Sultry. Complex. Serious. Gutsy. The brunette Bombshell is no pushover (see Tantrums, page 28). Hollywood brunettes have been known to pack a pistol (Jane Russell in *The Outlaw*), grind stilettos into a man's foot

(Elizabeth Taylor in *Butterfield 8*) and march across Spain for a cause (Sophia Loren in *The Pride and the Passion*). The brunette Bombshell is enigmatic. Mysterious. She never reveals her cards. She elicits questions. Fantasies. That doesn't mean she's not vulnerable. It's just not the first thing you see.

The Redheaded Bombshell

Red and auburn are not the first choices of the Bombshell. She doesn't want to be known as a carrot top or have anything to do with the garish color associated with clowns. The redheaded Bombshell has depth and heat. Think hot lava. Virtually uncharted territory, it takes a rare Bombshell to pull it off. One who is willing to self-invent. The redheaded Bombshell is vibrant, poised, enthusiastic like Rita Hayworth, whose acting style was described by choreographer Hermes Pan as developing from the inside out. "At first there is a terrifying stillness, then the dormant self wakes and there is a volcano." (See Tantrums, page 28.)

Bathing Caps

Bombshells wear bathing caps (exception: skinny dipping). Pool, lake or sea. Upon removing the cap—which will happen while still ankle deep and/or on the steps coming out of the pool—she will toss her head back and shake out her hair. Every Bombshell cultivates her own post-swim-head-shaking style.

BOMBSHELL BEAUTY

The Bombshell doesn't need expensive creams, lotions or serums. She believes in cold cream and soap. Marilyn Monroe washed her face several times a day with soap and water to keep her skin blemish free. Ava Gardner started out with Lava soap before converting to Neutrogena. That is not to say the Bombshell does not have her moments of extravagance. The bathtub, for instance. The Bombshell is a connoisseur. Champagne baths, ice baths, perfumed bubble baths, milk baths.

The Bombshell also swears by massage. She considers it part of her exercise regimen.

Bombshell Beauty Products

Camay or Dove or Ivory soap
Pond's cold cream
Vaseline
Noxzema
Bath oil beads

Jean Naté
Calgon
Johnson's Baby Shampoo (no more tears)
Prell
Pepsodent
Pearl Drops
Arpège or Chanel body talc and puff
Epsom salts

Makeup

While the Bombshell has no problem showing up or being discovered in various states of undress, she will never be seen without makeup. She wears it in bubble baths, she wears it to sleep. Bombshell makeup might look simple, but it's deceptively time intensive.[1] Eyelashes alone can take twenty minutes to affix. Highly stylized and in a limited palette, Bombshell makeup is never trendy, flashy or experimental.

The Bombshell values clean, scrubbed skin. She does not cover up with pancake or heavy foundation. If she uses it at all, she applies it lightly and then dabs most of it off (she may also use a cream foundation such as Almay) before dusting with T. LeClerc loose powder from the tin. She will have LeClerc powders in several colors including Orchidée, a luminous lavender pink, for evening. For her colors, she trusts the girl at the counter.

---

1 Elizabeth Taylor insisted on wearing makeup for every scene in *Cleopatra*, even when she was told she didn't need it, according to C. David Heymann in *Liz: An Intimate Biography of Elizabeth Taylor*. When caught dabbing powder on the roof of her mouth, she allegedly said, "Well, they'll see the inside of my mouth when I speak my lines. I want to look perfect."

Lipstick

A Bombshell does not cultivate an icy personality and, therefore, does not like frosted lipstick. She does, however, add a glaze or gloss over her lipstick. There are three Bombshell colors: pink, red and nude. The Bombshell generally specializes in one of these, but is not committed. Bombshells are famous for blending two to five shades at once. She may tell you she's wearing Cherries in the Snow, but there'll probably be a few other colors in the mix.

Pink

Pink is the baby-doll nightgown of lipsticks. Jayne Mansfield favored it. Lush, over-the-top bubblegum pink with the faintest hint of lilac. Bombshell pink is always a bit startling, never tamed by taupe or jazzed by sparkle. It has the audacious, no-apology quality of a pink Cadillac.

Favorites

Tibet by Christian Dior

Love That Pink by Revlon
(Not a whisper pink . . . a whistle pink)

Coco Pink by Chanel

Beautiful Pink by Estée Lauder

Witty Fuchsia by Estée Lauder

Pink Nouveau by M•A•C

Rouge Pur 49 by YSL

Red

Marilyn Monroe wore red. All Bombshells have red lipstick in their repertoire. Vibrant, obvious, seen-from-across-the-room red. Blue reds, red reds, orange reds—as long as it goes with her coloring. Never brick, copper, anything burnt, mapled or leaning toward brown. A Bombshell prefers a name with pizzazz.

The Bombshell treats red with respect. She does not brandish it for all occasions. While she might wear it horseback riding, she would never wear it to a funeral or any event where she might upstage her husband.

FAVORITES

Cherries in the Snow by Revlon
Fire and Ice by Revlon
Certainly Red by Revlon
Love That Red by Revlon
Holiday Red by Christian Dior
Dolce Vita by Christian Dior
Jungle Red by Nars
Red Star by Chanel
Slick Red by Estée Lauder
Rouge Pur Mat 5 by YSL
Rouge Pur 11 by YSL
Ruby Woo by M•A•C

Nude

Brigitte Bardot went nude. Kim Novak didn't like a loud mouth either. "I wear light and very little lipstick," she said. "But I'd feel naked without eye makeup. With the mouth, your words speak for you. But your eyes must express what's inside without words."

FAVORITES

Beige Mischief by Christian Dior
Cashmere by Christian Dior
Belle de Jour by Nars
Beige de Chanel by Chanel
In the Buff by Revlon
Hush by M•A•C

Eye Makeup

Bombshells have been known to emulate what Marilyn Monroe called "the Garbo eye," using a white shadow under the brow and shaping the lid with a bruised, natural-looking blend of blue and smoke, never flattening brown. Special occasions may call for liquid lilac or creamy silver. Sometimes Bombshells opt for a simple dusting of luminescent champagne, such as Nars's aptly named Bombshell, to set off diamonds or pearls.

Contemporary Bombshells often forgo eyeshadow altogether and stick to liner and lashes. Eyeliner will be black or brown, liquid or cake, swept across the lash line and out to a point. Bombshells do not reserve false eyelashes for special occasions but see them as a daily necessity like vitamins. For day she puts on small clusters of eyelashes, three to five in each, separated from a full set, possibly the ones she wore last night. She will apply these with clear eyelash glue using tweezers, primarily at the outer edges of the eye. Mascara is always black, waterproof of course—Chanel, Helena Rubenstein or Maybelline, the pink and green kind. Bombshells also use cake mascara and own eyelash curlers.

Eyebrows

The Bombshell likes well-shaped, well-endowed eyebrows. She sees them as an opportunity to create an expressive, poignant arch. Elizabeth Taylor is famous for her thoroughbred brows. Voluptuous, dense, dark and peaked, they are a dramatic counterpoint to her pale skin and violet eyes. Elizabeth Taylor's eyebrows say, *Stop, look at me. Look again.*

Bombshell eyebrow grooming tools include an eyebrow brush, pencils and powder color. She likes brow shaper powder by Elizabeth Arden and pencils by Maybelline.

A blonde Bombshell likes her brows a good shade or two darker than her hair.

Beauty Marks

Bombshells believe in them. Whether it's a true beauty mark or a freckle, a Bombshell plays it up with a little black pencil. She considers it evening wear appropriate for cocktail parties and black-tie events.

Nail Polish

Bombshells can take it or leave it. Red for fingers, coral for toes. Bombshells also wear clear. No French manicures. Bombshell nails are rounded, medium in length—never long, and always groomed.

The Bombshell in the Woods

The Bombshell loves natural landmarks. Old Faithful at Yellowstone National Park. The Grand Canyon. The Petrified Forest. She appreciates the novelty of a cabin in the woods (as long as there's a fireplace and a down comforter), horseback riding and an occasional hike.

When the Bombshell is in a rustic setting and over-the-top glamour is too much, she has ways of retaining Bombshell status. First, she never entirely lets go of the jewels, fake or real. She may place them more discreetly, in her hair, for example, or pare down to a simple bracelet. Rings never count. Makeup, eyelashes included, goes unaltered no matter how rugged the terrain, and she will opt for a lighter outdoorsy scent (see Perfume, page 50). But tailoring is what most concerns the Bombshell when going to the woods. Her dungarees (as she calls them) are fitted, and may be rolled a good two inches at the cuff. Her blouse, white, plaid or gingham cotton (his or hers), can be instantly modified by tying the fabric tight around the waist, cinched. Cool weather may call for chamois or flannel. Buttons are more decorative than useful since only one may be necessary with this method.

Should the Bombshell encounter a lake, she will, weather permitting and if the company is pleasing to her, go skinny dipping (see Bombshells in the Buff, page 44). The Bombshell on horseback wears boots with a heel. As for walking, there is no limit to how high heels can be. She knows how to walk in high heels, hell, she knows how to run in them. If, for some reason, she finds it difficult to navigate in high heels while hiking, she simply takes them off and carries them limply in her hand.

Cold Weather Tips

The Bombshell knows how to stay warm; she knows that it is most important to cover the head, hands and feet.[1] And since her feet are out of the question (open-toe sandals are a must, high heeled, of course) and a hat is not ever welcome (a chiffon or silk scarf will do), gloves are of the utmost importance. A Bombshell carries gloves with her from September through April. She knows that they are always a good prop and maintaining the softness of her hands is terribly important. The scarf is worn around the neck and draped down the back unless it is snowing, in which case the scarf will be worn on the head (see Scarves, page 68).

The Bombshell detests coats—even furs, shawls, wraps—she hates them all. She drapes them over her shoul-

---

1 Lurking in the back of the Bombshell's closet is a pair of ankle-high black felt boots lined with faux fur she bought on a trip to Vermont. She usually comes across them in the spring. Marilyn Monroe owned a pair, shown in Christie's catalogue, *The Personal Property of Marilyn Monroe*. They show remarkably little wear.

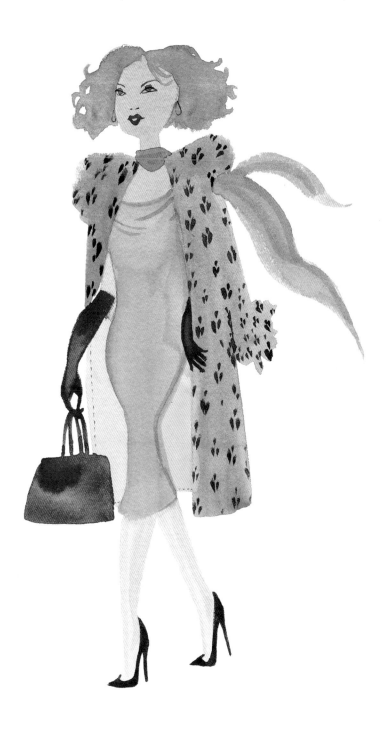

ders; she never puts her arms through the sleeves (see Elizabeth Taylor in *The Last Time I Saw Paris* or just about any Bombshell in any movie. Exception: Dramatic exits. Miss Taylor in *Butterfield 8* absconding with a full-length mink and almost nothing underneath).

Rainy Weather Tips

When heading out into a storm, the Bombshell wears a trench coat and her most resilient sandals. Never slickers and rubber boots, which she calls galoshes, unless she's on board *The Maid of the Mist* or traversing the catwalk under the spray of Niagara Falls.

The Bombshell finds a sudden thunderstorm thrilling. She appreciates the spontaneity of an impromptu drenching and doesn't mind if her white polka-dot dress turns transparent and clings to every curve. However, there are two things that concern the Bombshell in a downpour. First, her shoes. As the first drops splash, she will remove them and go barefoot. This goes for all locations from boardwalks to piazzas to Fifth Avenue.

The second concern is her makeup. Under no circumstances does the Bombshell want her face to get wet. She will cover her head with a scarf or magazine if no umbrella is present. Men have been known to walk several blocks out of their way to keep a Bombshell's head covered and she has

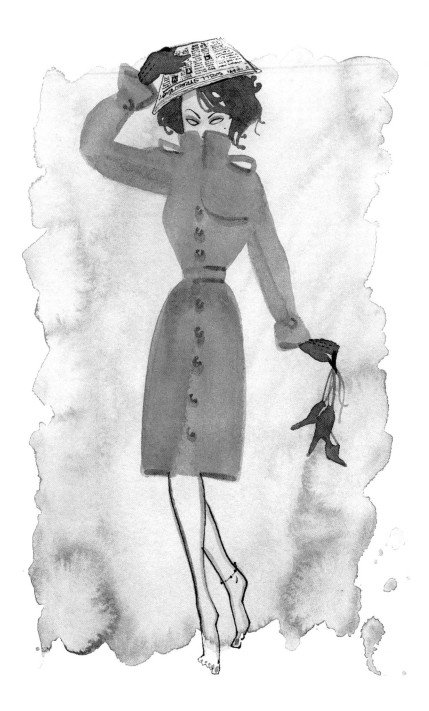

quite a collection of business cards to prove it (see The Bombshelter, The Kitchen, page 104).

As for umbrellas, she leaves them in cabs, finds them in cabs, takes the wrong one from the umbrella stand or forgets to take hers altogether. To the Bombshell, the umbrella is part of the universal recycling program.

III

Bombshell Lifestyle

Day-to-Day
Bombshellism

The Bombshell abhors routine. She is ready for anything at a moment's notice—a movie, a trip to Istanbul, a cocktail. She knows that a phone call can change her evening. Hell, it can change her life.

There is no such thing as a typical Bombshell day. She might wake up (to the *1812 Overture*; see Music, page 120), slip into her peignoir and matching mules, pull the manual typewriter from under the bed and work on her memoir for an hour, or until the phone rings.

If she feels like it, she may clean the bathroom tiles with an old toothbrush before taking a shower. Sometimes the downstairs neighbor, a playwright, brings her coffee. Otherwise, she has it delivered. She intends to buy an espresso maker, someday. Then she could make the playwright coffee for a change. She doesn't mind reading his plays. She's flattered, in fact. But the Bombshell can't understand why he always wants her to be the tramp or the showgirl, never the girl next door—besides, how can she expect her to act without pay in that basement on the Lower East Side or that awful place upstairs with no elevator?

On the way to the pastry shop the Bombshell will either:

A pop in for a manicure (she never makes an appointment)
B buy lingerie
C try out new perfumes, or
D pick up a copy of the latest *Variety, Vanity Fair* or *The New Yorker.*

Chances are, she'll end up having oysters for lunch at an outdoor cafe. (Unless she's in L.A. Then, reluctantly and only because Schwab's is no more, she'll go to the Coffee Bean and Tea Leaf at Sunset Plaza, never Starbucks.) No matter what her budget, you'll never find her at a fast-food joint. (Diners don't count, she finds them charming.) She'd rather have one small, exquisite meal in keeping with her fantasy life than spend her money practically, by stocking the cupboard. If, by coincidence, she's sitting next to a student with a university bulletin, she might ask for the page with the phone numbers. She's always wanted to take an art appreciation class.

It's likely, if she's unemployed, she'll make a call about work at this point—has a job come through? Did she get the job? Did she get the part?

A Bombshell is always in character (see Makeup, page 83). You will never find her commuting in running shoes with socks over nylons. She has too much self-esteem. To a Bombshell, a girl wearing unglamorous shoes in public is saying, "I hate myself, this part of my life doesn't count. I resent the shoes I am supposed to wear at work and besides, they're not comfortable and I am not interested in men." For a Bombshell, nothing is unimportant, nothing is impossible. She lives in anticipation of opportunity. That agent, photographer or future husband could be in the next elevator.

Even at home alone, a Bombshell is always glamorous.[1] She may change her clothing several times throughout the day, depending on her mood. When her favorite Frank Sinatra music program comes on, for example, she will often be moved to put on a cocktail dress. She never plans an outfit in advance. (Exclusions include special events like singing at presidential birthdays.) Needless to say, a Bombshell is always wearing perfume. She does this not to charm the occasional FedEx or FTD delivery man, but for her own pleasure. The Bombshell's idea of at-home casual wear may indeed be casual, but it's never sloppy. A Bombshell might do her laundry in a sexy black slip, but never sweatpants. A typical around-the-house lounging-on-the-couch outfit might be a sleeveless lamé top and leopard Capri pants or Chinese silk pajamas if it's after eight. Even in the privacy of her bathtub, a Bombshell has her hair loftily piled—never a shower cap—and will be wearing enough eye makeup to answer the door if necessary.

Most of all, a Bombshell enjoys her own company. She is not afraid to be alone. She will go to the Palm Court at the Plaza simply to entertain herself or to the top of the Seattle Space Needle for a cocktail at the revolving restaurant. A Bombshell loves a good view. Besides, she's effervescent, so a Bombshell is never alone for long.

1 In a newspaper interview Dolores Del Rio revealed, "If I am resting at home, I will wear perhaps some hostess pajamas or some simple housedress. Slacks? Never! I abominate them—they are not even comfortable. I like feminine things. And I could not be one of those women who must hurry to dress up when unexpected callers arrive. I love to dress—for myself."

THE BOMBSHELTER

The Bathroom

The bathroom is where the Bombshell spends most of her time.[1] Specifically, the bathtub. She does a variety of things here: works on her taxes, reads over her contracts, writes letters—business and personal—and most importantly, talks on the phone. Like her shoes, the Bombshell telephone is white, ivory, taupe or pink and occasionally light blue. It is never red, brown or black and always has a twenty-foot cord (never cordless). It is implicit that the phone match every room in her home. The bathroom itself is white or pink with black trim and features a plush rug. The Bombshell robe, or shall we say wardrobe of robes, includes at least one in white or champagne silk with matching marabou trim and a white cotton terry robe, extra big and sporting a hotel monogram.

Every Bombshell has the following things in her medicine cabinet: Band-Aids (essential for breaking in new

---

1 Jayne Mansfield had thirteen bathrooms in her mansion, the Pink Palace, on Sunset Boulevard.

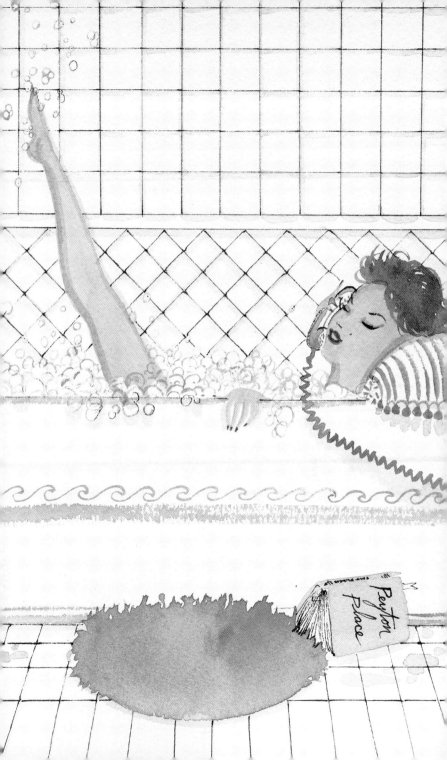

slingbacks), Aqua Net Extra Super Hold, Visine, Valium, Vaseline, baby aspirin, calamine lotion, eyelash adhesive, lavender smelling salts, three kinds of bobby pins, a first-aid kit that's never been opened and a miniature Eiffel Tower souvenir from Paris, France.

The Kitchen

The Bombshell refrigerator is a sort of vanity on ice and is primarily used to store nail polish, perfume and a bright blue eye mask. The maraschino cherries left over from a cocktail party sit next to a bottle of Chanel No. 19. Capers, olives and a magnum of Dom Pérignon are the only other nutritional substances in the Bombshell refrigerator. It is safe to say that she has never turned on the oven where she stores the pans given to her by a well-meaning great aunt. In the freezer we find plenty of ice, stockings in nude, suntan and black, a half-eaten carton of rum raisin ice cream and a bottle of Scandinavian vodka brought over by a composer friend who comes to her house for advice on Thursday nights.

The refrigerator door is the Bombshell's desk and Rolodex. This is where she keeps scraps of paper, a picture of herself posing with a small animal, postcards and business cards. It is understood that the business cards are purely for reference. The only man a Bombshell has ever considered calling was the young investment analyst with whom she shared a cab. She thought it was adorable that he took her seriously when she said she didn't have a diversified portfolio, that she only had one head shot.

The Bedroom

The Bombshell's bed of choice is, of course, a queen. The headboard is either smoked mirror, white faux bamboo, Florentine wood or quilted and upholstered in ivory-colored silk. Several throw pillows in shades that complement the room's color scheme are found here. A black silk bedspread, for example, might have several pink satin pillows strewn across it. These, of course, match the carpeting and drapes.

The Bombshell favors white Louis XV and XVI–style furniture with the occasional piece in Regency style. Her vanity, a large, white French-looking piece of furniture, doubles as a writing desk and the memoirs she started are in a top drawer. Favorite love letters are kept in a Tiffany box or tied with a pink ribbon. She keeps the rest under the bed in shoe boxes, preferably Manolo Blahnik. If a Bombshell has an alarm clock we have yet to see it. She relies on friends and wake-up services. She is never deliberately late (exception: Elizabeth Taylor).

Satin always figures in a Bombshell bedroom. Satin sheets (never flannel), quilted satin bedspread, bed jacket, curtains, slips, slippers, undergarments galore. A Bombshell celebrates her sensuality in the bedroom and views wall-to-wall carpeting as a lush necessity. She can't bear to step onto cold wood. Carpeting is moderately plush and may be pink, white, champagne or baby blue and often matches the telephone. The television, and the Bombshell always has one, is generally in the bedroom. Though she would lead you to believe she falls asleep reading, in truth the Bombshell watches old black-and-white movies and/or the weather man. Never nature films (see Tantrums, page 28).

Light is an enemy of Bombshell sleep. Therefore, Bombshell curtains are of the substantial variety, commonly known as blackout drapes, with a layer of sheer gauze floating underneath. Her interior decorator friend knew just what to bring over. It is not uncommon for a Bombshell's drapery to match one of her dresses.

Every Bombshell worth her salt has a decorative folding screen of white bamboo, Chinese painted wood or gilded wrought iron. To the Bombshell, no screen is complete without something intimate hanging over it.

There is always a little night table with a lamp next to the bed. This lamp will either be very tiny or very large, nothing in between. The lampshade will be covered with either dotted Swiss or silk shantung and have a ruffled edge. Some Bombshells have matching night tables on either side of the bed, in which case there will be matching lamps. The Lucite Kleenex box will hold tissues, scented, matching the color scheme, (i.e., white or pink, which comes in handy when she breaks down and watches the nature film after all—it seemed so cute in the beginning).

There is also a chandelier, unless the ceiling is too low, then she'll have one or two wall fixtures of cut glass. Her night-light is a seashell.

There will usually be a pink or mirrored dresser somewhere in the room, possibly in the walk-in closet. She may have had this since childhood. If the bedroom is large enough there will be an overstuffed chair or chaise longue. A Bombshell will sometimes entertain here.

There is no artwork in the Bombshell bedroom. That goes in the living room.

One last thing about beds. If a Bombshell wants to sleep under the stars, cots and sleeping bags are out of the question. Jane Russell had a big bed moved into the garden.

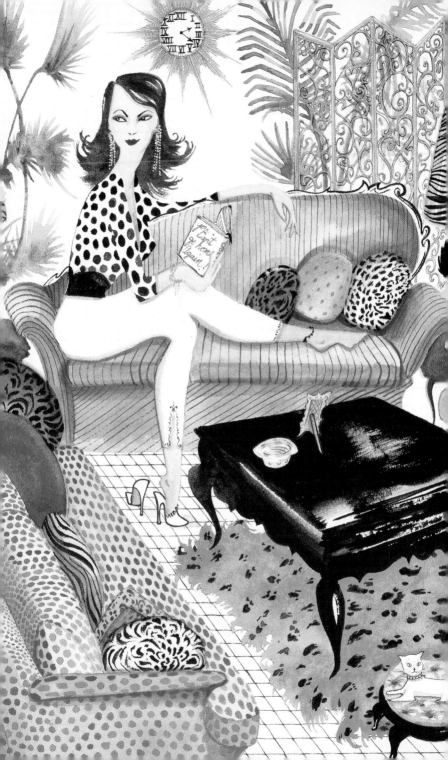

The Living Room

Every Bombshell has a piano in her living room, usually white, space permitting. Grand, baby grand, upright, it doesn't matter. At any moment, a gentleman caller may spontaneously compose a few bars for her—about her. There may be an Oriental vase on the piano. If it's not there, it's somewhere else in the room, probably on the fireplace mantel where you will also find a decorative clock. There is always a chandelier and a Chinese folding screen or two. (You never know when she'll run behind it and slip into something else.) When it comes to table lamps, the Bombshell prefers Tiffany or something Oriental. If she goes the Oriental route it will inevitably resemble one she saw in the lobby of a grand hotel, old movie or the living room of her music appreciation teacher when he invited the class over for wine—his wife wasn't very friendly.

Bombshell furniture is lacquered, French or Regency style. Her stereo goes in a marble-topped console and is stacked with Bombshell classics (see Music, page 120).

There will be a curvaceous, upholstered sofa in a solid color or leopard print. In any case, we're likely to find several leopard print pillows or a leopard print ottoman. Zebra will also do. The living room color theme will either be pink (Dorothy Dandridge/Jayne Mansfield) or white (Elizabeth Taylor/Marilyn Monroe).

A Bombshell wants her guests to feel at home and will therefore always have several souvenir ashtrays on the coffee table (mirrored or glass), including one from San Francisco or Niagara Falls. Matches are collected purely for sentimental reasons, never used. Her guests light up with a heavy cut-glass and ormolu lighter in the shape of a fruit, preferably a pineapple.

The living room is where the Bombshell showcases her art collection. It usually consists of two to three Impressionist paintings, a Vincent van Gogh, a Modigliani, a Spanish painter or two, at least one painting of an animal and a bust of Venus. There will also be many photographs of the Bombshell in small frames throughout the room, at least one of her cuddling an animal (there's another on the refrigerator). Paintings are often framed in gold—that way they match the gilt mirrors, of which there are several.

Ten Things You Will Never Find in a Bombshell Home

1 Taxidermy (exceptions: bear rugs for pets to sleep on and anything shot or caught by her lover/husband.)
2 Fly swatters
3 Pot holders
4 Fluorescent lights
5 Nautical anything
6 Drawer of coupons/receipts/rubber bands
7 Unbreakable plates and glasses
8 Coffee mugs with cute expressions and/or pictures
9 Sticky traps
10 Calculators

The Bombshell Library

The Bombshell's library doesn't always merit a room of its own. In fact, her collection may consist entirely of books on the floor surrounding her bed or stacked so that she can, say, climb up on them to, say, open a window. If the Bombshell in question does actually have a library proper, while giving a tour of her home she might say something like, "This is where it all happens." She knows that to be an attractive woman is one thing, to be beautiful is another, and that to be a Bombshell it takes brains—maybe not the mathematical or scientific kind, but a Bombshell is at least mildly conversant in matters physiological, poetic and philosophical. And, of course, she has at least one annotated history book which doubles as an ottoman.

It is understood that the Bombshell's library has an eclectic nature. We would not be surprised to find a text-book on physics next to *The Great Gatsby*. However, the appearance of a textbook usually indicates that it is either a gift or suggested reading by someone in particular, probably an older man (see inside for telltale inscription). It is not impossible to find a Bombshell reading up on mc² and quantum physics, but it is unlikely. The Bombshell's library includes gifts, overdue library books and inheritances. But she plans on reading them all. It's just a matter of when!

As for the books she picks out for herself, the Bombshell likes an author who writes about someone like her (with compassion, of course). This is not out of vanity, but rather because she feels misunderstood. Books about women like her teach her something about herself, about how to be herself, although it is important to realize that this is not narcissism but something more complicated and innocent. She adores Jack Kerouac and the all-American convertible-driving blondes he meets along the way. She can relate to a man like Sal Paradise or Cody; they express the wanderlust she feels, too, but can't put into words. She is on her own road.

What She Carries

Thomas Wolfe's *You Can't Go Home Again* (Her favorite, it makes her cry, she knows she can't go home again. What's even sadder is that she feels she has no home.)

Nietzsche's *Thus Spake Zarathustra A Book for All and None* (She feels she has the same questions about life as

Nietzsche. At least she thinks so from the four pages she's read. It gave her nightmares.)

What's on Her Shelf

Oscar Wilde's *Salome*

Marcel Proust's *Remembrance of Things Past*

Grace Metalious's *Peyton Place* (She saw Jayne Mansfield reading this in a bubble bath in a movie.)

Gore Vidal's *Lincoln* and *Hollywood*

Gentlemen Prefer Blondes and everything else by Anita Loos

Colette's *The Complete Claudine* (A gift from a French literature scholar she met in a pastry shop.)

Shakespeare's *Sonnets* (Library book, three years overdue.)

Shakespeare's *Antony and Cleopatra*

George Bernard Shaw's *Caesar and Cleopatra*

Bartlett's Familiar Quotations (She would carry this around but it's too heavy.)

The Bible (Taken from a motel.)

Henry Miller's Trilogy: *Sexus, Nexus, Plexus* (A gift.)

Plato's *Republic*

Sigmund Freud's *Character and Culture* (Analyst's suggestion.)

Kahlil Gibran's *The Prophet* (She used to carry this around.)

Bulfinch's Mythology (Consistently being compared to goddesses, she wants to investigate this further.)

The Giant Golden Book of Elves and Fairies

Walt Whitman's *Leaves of Grass* (Water-damaged from propping open windows.)

D. H. Lawrence's *Women in Love* (Water-damaged from being dropped in the tub.)

Arthur Schopenhauer's *The World as Will and Representation*

(Rita Hayworth gives Schopenhauer the Bombshell seal of approval by singing about him in *Pal Joey*.)
Rumi
The Speeches of Abraham Lincoln and various presidential biographies
Watty Piper's *The Little Engine That Could* (She reads this when she needs to rev up her courage.)
Antoine de Saint-Exupéry's *The Little Prince*
F. Scott Fitzgerald's *The Great Gatsby*
The Astrology Handbook
French in 10 Days
Italian in 10 Days

She has a special section on her shelf for books about animals and wildlife:

Jack London, canon
Moby-Dick
Animal Farm
The Yearling
Watership Down
Pat the Bunny
Edith and the Bears
Koko's Kitten

What She Does Not Have and Has Not Read

J. D. Salinger (The "Bananafish" thing makes her queasy.)
William Faulkner (Just too sad.)
Carl Jung

Joseph Campbell

Robert Bly

Emily Dickinson (Her lack of sex appeal is charming but she's just too morose.)

Henry Thoreau

Mark Twain

Ralph Waldo Emerson

Marquis de Sade

T. S. Eliot

Sylvia Plath (She thought Sylvia was pretty, picked up a volume in a bookstore but when she read the intro about her suicide, put it down. Similarly, she decided not to read a book of Anne Sexton's poems—another beautiful poet—when she heard the story about her hugging an air conditioner in her analyst's office.)

Virginia Woolf (She saw Elizabeth Taylor in the movie and doesn't want to know anything about that woman.)

Henry James

John Steinbeck's *Of Mice and Men* (She can appreciate a man not knowing his own strength but she heard about the puppies and the rabbits and doesn't understand why the guy's brother didn't just give him a stuffed animal.)

Arthur Rimbaud

Samuel Beckett

And especially John Updike

Bombshell Handwriting

There are two varieties of Bombshell handwriting: public and private. The Bombshell has been practicing public penmanship—autographs, *X*'s and *O*'s and thank-you's—since childhood, dashing off flamboyant, curly, voluptuous letters in yearbooks, on note pads, napkins and school papers. Her first initials always dominate the page and it is generally understood that the signature optimistically slants upward at roughly 45 degrees. Dolores Del Rio liked to take up the whole page.[1]

The Bombshell takes every opportunity to fill out "this notebook belongs to." Every document signed is an autograph, to the Bombshell—from a lease to a pet license to a

---

1 "She's an autograph seeker's delight," a Hollywood reporter wrote, "because she loves to sign them and when she hands the pen back to one of the hounds it's usually dry. For regardless of the size of the piece of paper presented for her signature, she covers it with her name. Dolores figures if they want her signature, she'll really give them one."

photo release.[2] Bombshells have been know to dot their *i*'s with a heart or rhinestone (in cement) and finish their signature with a lip print.

The telephone will always be the first means of communication for the Bombshell, but she does write thank-you letters and will rewrite them several times if she's made a mistake or if the handwriting isn't neat and curvaceous enough, no matter how expensive the stationery. The Bombshell knows that any written correspondence may have a future life in a library, in a book or in *People* magazine.

Private handwriting, i.e., poetry, shopping lists, diary entries, on the other hand is candid, vulnerable, *au naturel*. She may be wearing mules while writing her shaky little shopping list, but her handwriting will betray whatever she's feeling that day. Let it be known that the Bombshell may have had a considerable amount of champagne before making an entry in her diary, which will have an effect on her penmanship. Mascara and salty tears may also add to the emotional texture of the page.

2 Dominick Dunne, who interviewed Ava Gardner for *Vanity Fair* in 1984, wrote, "In a magical star gesture, a throwback to her MGM days, she signed the photo release form as if she were bestowing an autograph at a premiere."

BOMBSHELL STATIONERY

The Bombshell is enamored with her initials. She will take every opportunity to have them printed, engraved and embossed on her stationery supplies. These include 8½-by-11-inch and 4-by-6-inch lined notepaper with initials on the upper left corner (she only uses the small one), engraved notecards with her initials in pink or gold on white, or black or gold on pink. Bombshells have been known to add their husbands' last initial to their own.[1] Sooner or later, every Bombshell breaks down and has her whole name engraved. The stationery consultant (at Dempsey & Carrol, Tiffany or Cartier) may subtly try to dissuade her from colors used exclusively for baby announcements, but this has the opposite effect. The Bombshell will also have cards made or purchase ready-made cards with pineapples, bees, small fluffy dogs or fleur-de-lis. These are never in pink. That would not be sophisticated. The Bombshell also collects stationery from

1 Upon marrying Arthur Miller, Marilyn Monroe added another *M* to her two.

hotels. It all goes in a red leather case with her initials engraved in gold.

Pens are another story. The Bombshell has been given numerous Tiffany ballpoint pens in pastel colors sprinkled with a few Mont Blanc fountain pens. She also has a vast collection of No. 2 pencils—she has no idea where they've come from—which she uses to dial or press the buttons on her telephone.

Despite this ample collection, the Bombshell is always asking, "Do you have a pen?" There might be one in the bag that goes with the polka-dot sundress, but today she's wearing pink Pucci. That's a different handbag altogether. And how is she supposed to remember to buy those tiny little ink cartridges?

A Bombshell scents her correspondence indiscriminately. Gas company bills, contracts, postcards, she spritzes the whole mail heap—love letters get special attention. However, the Bombshell is not as frivolous with her lip prints as one might think. They are reserved for her current lover, husband and veterinarian, unless she's Kim Novak and husband and veterinarian are one and the same.

Things the Bombshell Monograms

Towels

Luggage

Bathrobes

Cotton and/or silk nightshirts and nightgowns

Linen handkerchiefs

Things the Bombshell
Monograms for Him

Slippers

Pajamas

Shirts

Bombshell Music

Schooled in the nuances of atmosphere, the Bombshell puts her faith in her stereo. She knows that music should never be too distracting, yet it should leave a lasting impression. A Bombshell treats her music like perfume. She is very selective and sophisticated in her musical preferences. And while she is indeed spontaneous, she does not leave her soundtrack to happenstance. While waiting for the bell to ring she rifles through her favorite classics—the sad ladies of jazz, the crooners, the French heartbreakers, the loud lively men—looking for a tune to create the right climate. For instance, if her neighbor is stopping by in the morning with coffee, she will play something optimistic like Louis Armstrong's "What a Wonderful World." (Keep in mind, she woke up to the *1812 Overture*.) For a distressed girlfriend, she might start with Carmen McRae and progress to Maria Callas. And she's too smart to play anything classical for an evening with a tightly wound financial analyst. She knows the innocent, smooth, tactile singing of Astrud Gilberto (*"The Girl from Ipanema"*) will disarm, and will, in fact, virtually unbutton him. It is not unheard of for the Bombshell's visitor to inquire with great urgency, "Who is that we're listening to?"

The Bombshell always knows what music will go with what outfit. She gets dressed up for Frank Sinatra, every Bombshell's favorite. Out comes the rhinestone bracelet, even if she's alone. There is a 50 percent chance that when a Bombshell answers the phone, Frank Sinatra will be on in the background. A full-bodied composer like Beethoven complements a black or white ensemble. Tchaikovsky is ideal for plunging necklines in red and deep shades of pink. Her favorite operas, *Madama Butterfly*, *La Bohème*, *Aida* and *Carmen,* inspire her to go over the top: kimonos, golden sheaths, showgirl velvet underscored with a corset.

Tito Puente, Xavier Cugat and Chico O'Farrill are opportunities to dress up in peasant blouses that slope off the shoulder, bangle bracelets, huge hoop earrings and skirts slit to there (think designers Tracy Feith and Anna Sui). Music of this sort calls for strappy high heels in bright or metallic colors. The Bombshell couldn't agree more with that fashion doyenne Diana Vreeland, who said, "A little bad taste is like a nice splash of paprika."

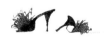

Within every Bombshell there lurks a little cornball. She adores the cha–cha, rhumba and, much to every-one's surprise, polka. She loves nothing more than to kick up her heels alone while sipping a little champagne. Bombshells often include singing and ukulele playing among their talents.[1,2,3]

Let it be known that the Bombshell never stoops to the top twenty or anything too predictable.

The Twenty-Four-Hour Bombshell Soundtrack

RISE AND SHINE

Peter I. Tchaikovsky, *1812 Overture*
Ludwig van Beethoven, *9th Symphony*
Glenn Miller, "In the Mood"

---

1 Brigitte Bardot and Serge Gainsbourg recorded "Bonnie and Clyde" as well as the risqué tunes "Harley David Son of a Bitch" and the legendary "Je t'aime . . . Moi Non Plus" (translation: *I love you . . . me neither.*) This particular collaboration, a suggestive little number punctuated by lots of heavy breathing, so outraged Bardot's then-husband, Gunther Sachs, that Gainsbourg withdrew it from sale and later re-recorded it with his lover Jane Birkin. Brigitte Bardot also recorded several albums on her own including the self-titled *Brigitte Bardot* and *Initials B.B.*

2 Bette Davis, in her southern, platinum-haired Bombshell role in *The Cabin in the Cotton*, clearly can't hold a note and sings flat but radiates sensual, kitten appeal like nobody's business.

3 Marilyn Monroe had her first piano lessons when she was five. Although never proficient, her performance of "Chopsticks" in the film *The Seven Year Itch* was done perfectly in only one take. Marilyn plays ukulele in *Some Like It Hot* and the guitar in *River of No Return,* where she is also a saloon singer. She sang in no less than ten movies/musicals, including *Let's Make Love* and sang for the American troops in Korea, and let's not forget that she sang "Happy Birthday" to JFK.

Scott Joplin, "Maple Leaf Rag"
Les Brown and His Orchestra, "Leap Frog"

Morning Exercise (Floor or Shower)

Robert Mitchum, "Momma Looka Boo Boo" (so much
cuter than Harry Belafonte's rendition)
Xavier Cugat, "Mambo No. 5"
Ella Fitzgerald/Louis Armstrong/ Eartha Kitt, "Let's Do It"
Frank Sinatra, "Come Fly with Me"

Morning Grooming

Edvard Grieg, *Peer Gynt Suite*
Maria Callas, hand-picked selections from *Carmen*
Glenn Miller, "Sunrise Serenade"
Johann Sebastian Bach, *Suite No. 1 in G major* (for eyelash and
eyeliner application)

Morning Coffee (with Neighbor)

Louis Armstrong, "What a Wonderful World"
Peggy Lee, "Black Coffee"
Nina Simone, "Sugar in My Bowl"
Frank Sinatra, "Blue Skies"

Bubble Bath

Camille Saint-Saëns, "Aquarium" and "The Swan"
Peter I. Tchaikovsky, "Dance of the Sugar Plum Fairy"
Maria Callas, *La Wally:* "Ebben? ne andrò lontanna"

DRESSING — FESTIVE COLORS

Milton Nascimento, "O Cavaleiro"
Chico O'Farrill, "Momentumi"
Xavier Cugat, "One Mint Julep"
Cachao, "Mambo"

DRESSING — SOMBER MOODS

Françoise Hardy, "Suzanne"
Ella Fitzgerald, "Cry Me a River" (alternative: Sam Cooke
    version)

DRESSING — SEQUINS, LAMÉ, SKIN-TIGHT GOWNS

Glenn Miller, "Moonlight Cocktail"
Frank Sinatra, "I've Got You Under My Skin"

DRESSING — DUNGAREES, PLAID SHIRTS FOR HIKES, ETC.

Les Paul and Mary Ford, "Hummingbird"

DRESSING FOR SHOPPING

Sarah Vaughan, "It's De-Lovely"
Blossom Dearie, "Always True to You in My Fashion"
Louis Armstrong, "Ain't Misbehavin'"
The Mills Brothers, "I Found a Million Dollar Baby (In a
    Five and Ten Cent Store)"

Pining Away

Yves Montand, "La Vie en Rose"
Chet Baker, "My Funny Valentine" and canon

Dancing (Alone or with a Partner)

Glenn Miller, "String of Pearls"
Benny Goodman, "Sing, Sing, Sing"
Artie Shaw, "It Ain't Right," "Thou Swell," "All the Things You Are," "Begin the Beguine," "Frenesi," "Moonglow"
Chico O'Farrill, "Chico's Cha Cha Cha"
Nat "King" Cole, "For Sentimental Reasons" (slow dance)

Waiting for the Doorbell to Ring

Etta James, "At Last"
Peggy Lee, "Fever"
Françoise Hardy, "Parlez-moi de lui"
Frank Sinatra, "Moon River"
Ella Fitzgerald, "Night and Day"
Maria Callas, from *Carmen*: "L'amour est un Oiseau Rebelle"

Cocktails

Count Basie and His Orchestra, "April in Paris"
Ella Fitzgerald, "'S Wonderful"
Yves Montand, "C'est Si Bon"
Francis Lai, "A Man and a Woman"
Eartha Kitt, "Je Cherche un Homme"

DIM THE LIGHTS

Fred Astaire, "I Concentrate on You"
Billy Eckstein, "In the Still of the Night"
Louis Armstrong and Oscar Peterson, "You Go to My Head"
Nat "King" Cole, "Blue Gardenia"
Glenn Miller, "Moonlight Serenade"
Ludwig van Beethoven, "Moonlight Sonata"
Tony Bennett, "Wrap Your Troubles in Dreams (and Dream Your Troubles Away)"
Oscar Peterson Plays Duke Ellington, "Lady of the Lavender Mist"
Carmen McRae, "I Only Have Eyes for You"

HEARTBREAK

Bing Crosby, "Me and the Moon"
Bing Crosby, "Ol' Man River"
Frédéric Chopin, Prelude in D flat major, opus 28 #15, "Raindrops"
Maria Callas, from *Madama Butterfly*: "Un Bel dì Vedremo"

BEDTIME

Harry James, "Sleepy Lagoon"
Frank Sinatra, "In the Wee Small Hours"
Ella Fitzgerald, "Dream a Little Dream of Me"

ANYTIME

Stan Getz/João Gilberto/Astrud Gilberto, "Girl from Ipanema"

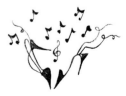

Bombshell
Diet & Beverages

Any Bombshell will tell you that she eats, not out of unhappiness, but out of joy. Nonpareils, sugared fruit slices, marshmallows, cotton candy, cherry pie, caviar, hot dogs, hamburgers, potato chips, salami sandwiches, chocolate-covered cherries and chocolate-covered anything are among the Bombshell's favorite foods. Calories are not an issue. When teased about her appetite, Sophia Loren said, "Everything you see I owe to spaghetti."

This does not mean the Bombshell has no regard for health and diet. She's eaten her share of cottage cheese, yogurt, wheat germ and grapefruit, but only when she's on a kick or needs to drop a few pounds. When it comes to dieting, the Bombshell seeks guidance. She calls her doctor and when he won't give her any more of those pills, she tries the recommended menu. (See Marilyn Monroe's diet plan, pages 136–37.) Bombshells have also been known to check themselves in.

The Bombshell likes to read up on health trends and will have pamphlets like *Kelp and Honey* in the drawer where she keeps the corkscrew. She does not eat tofu or drink wheatgrass. If she has a juicer, and there's a 50 percent chance she does, there's a 100 percent chance she's never used it.

The Bombshell is a liberated woman. She enjoys being a sex object and feels virtually no pressure to have culinary prowess. Jane Russell's husband, Bob Waterfield, told a magazine writer that he did the cooking in their home because he saw no point in Jane bending over a hot stove and, maybe, "scorching her career." However, that does not mean the Bombshell doesn't take a stab at cooking, or have at least one recipe up her sleeve. Jane Russell once recited her recipe for Green Pepper Steak à la Waterfield, suspiciously named after the real cook in her household.

Household appliances not traditionally used for cooking show up in the Bombshell kitchen.

When describing her eggplant recipe to the *New York Post*, Sophia Loren said, "The secret is to take all the bitterness out of the eggplant. You cut them up and put a weight on them—like an iron or something—to remove the bitterness."

Marilyn Monroe told *Cosmopolitan* that when making homemade noodles for a dinner party, the cookbook failed to mention how long they took to dry. "The guests arrived; I gave them a drink; I said, 'You have to wait for dinner until the noodles dry. Then we'll eat.' I had to give them another drink. In desperation, I went and got my little portable hair dryer and turned it on. It blew the noodles off the counter, and I had to gather them up and try again."

Do not be deceived by the ragged condition of the cookbooks found in the Bombshell's kitchen. These include *Fanny Farmer's Cook Book* and *The New Joy of Cooking,* and possibly *Amy Vanderbilt's Complete Cookbook* and the *Betty Crocker Cookbook*. Usually she has inherited these books.

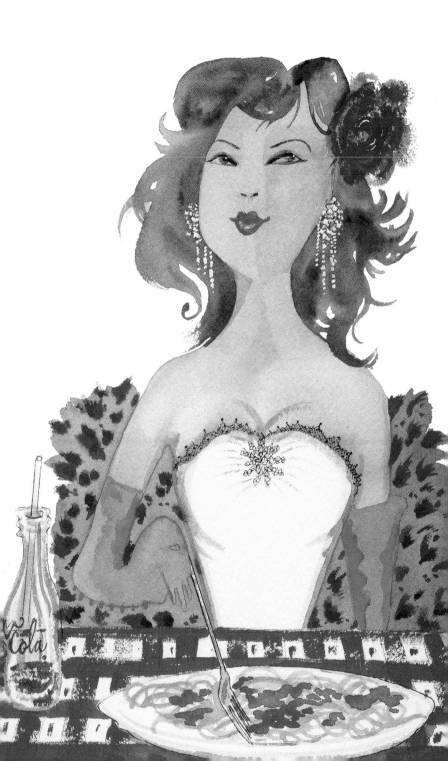

Aunts. Neighbors. Friends. She peruses them with good intentions. She has marked the following recipes: Pineapple Upside Down Cake, Cream Puffs, Chocolate Soufflé and Angel Food Cake. The only one she's tried out so far is Ambrosia.

The Bombshell likes a dessert with a big presentation. Crêpes Suzette, Baked Alaska, Bananas Flambé—anything liquored up and ignited or à la mode.

The Bombshell also likes a dish with a title: Lobster à la Newburg, Fettuccini Leon, Lobster à la Delmonico, Oysters à la D'Uxelles, Oysters Rockefeller, Beef Wellington, Waldorf Salad.

When a Bombshell caters her own party, she serves small food such as canapés, cherry tomatoes (Marilyn Monroe's favorite appetizer was tiny tomatoes stuffed with cream cheese and caviar), pearl onions, egg rolls, deviled eggs, mushroom caps, shrimp cocktail, fondue, cubed salami and cheese with cocktail toothpicks, Swedish meatballs and pigs in a blanket. The most beloved of Bombshell party recipes involve not cooking but assembly, which may take a while. (Many Bombshells have never used their oven.) Someone always offers to run out and buy the eggs and other miscellaneous ingredients. The Bombshell keeps serving drinks until the small food is prepared. That is, until someone finally comes into the kitchen and helps. The Bombshell is not lazy. Being a sensitive person, she is generally more concerned with entertaining than cooking.

Favorite Bombshell Entertaining Recipes

PIGS IN A BLANKET (FROZEN)

Follow directions on box.

AMBROSIA
(The Bombshell's personal variation)

2 large Valencia oranges
3 ripe bananas
1 can pineapple chunks
¼ cup confectioner's sugar
1½ cups shredded coconut
1 cup miniature marshmallows
¼ cup whole maraschino cherries (stemmed and pitted)

Mix well in a bowl. Chill before serving in individual parfait cups. Garnish with whipped cream.

STRAWBERRIES LIBERTÉ
(From the Club Alabam in Chicago, circa 1958)

Select the biggest, firmest ripe strawberries available. Cut a small slice from the tip so that the berry may stand upright.

With a demitasse spoon or a narrow, sharp knife or both, hollow out the stem of each berry and fill the cavities with fresh caviar. Stand each berry on a slice of lime and sprinkle with vodka. The very smallest glass jar of caviar will take care of 6 large strawberries.

Anchovy Canapés
(From the aunt from Florida with all the wigs)

Spread triangular pieces of toasted bread with anchovy butter from the gourmet shop. Hard boil eggs or ask someone
to bring these. Separate the yolks and whites and chop sepa-
rately. Cover half of each canapé with chopped yolk, and half
with chopped whites. Separate yolk from white with an
anchovy. If there's time, pipe around a border of anchovy
butter. Do this very carefully with a small knife or really do
it right with a pastry bag and tube. Borrow one from the
lady across the street.

Caviar Dip Extravaganza

Mix ½ cup Reddi-wip or real whipped cream with ½ ounce
caviar in a crystal bowl. Center on a platter and surround
with celery sticks and triangles of rye toast.

Tomatoes Stuffed with Caviar
(The Bombshell had these at a movie producer's house)

12 cherry tomatoes
6 tablespoons caviar
1 small bar cream cheese
chives

Slice off top and scoop out the center of the tomatoes. Place a
dollop of cream cheese in each tomato and top with caviar.
Garnish with chives. Chill before serving.

Shrimp Cocktail
(This is the Bombshell's personal recipe)

Use deveined, cooked shrimp. Chill thoroughly. To serve, arrange petite lettuce leaves in individual seafood cocktail glasses or dessert dishes (borrow these from a neighbor). Curve shrimp around edges. Garnish with lemon slices. The cocktail sauce goes in a separate bowl. If there's time, make one of those cocktail sauces from a cookbook.

Cuban Cocktail Sauce

3 to 6 tablespoons chili sauce
2 tablespoons horseradish
A squeeze of lemon juice
$\frac{1}{2}$ teaspoon salt
$\frac{1}{8}$ teaspoon pepper
A pinch of cayenne pepper
1 splash Worcestershire sauce
2 splashes Tabasco sauce
1 splash cognac (Champagne will do in a pinch.)

Mix well and chill.

New Orleans Cocktail Sauce

$\frac{1}{3}$ cup salad oil
2 tablespoons wine vinegar
2 tablespoons paprika
2 tablespoons mustard
2 tablespoons chopped parsley
2 minced green onions
2 tablespoons chopped celery

¹/₂ teaspoon salt
¹/₈ teaspoon pepper

Mix all ingredients and chill.

Fondue

(4 servings)

Grate: 1 lb. Emmenthaler or ¹/₂ lb. Emmenthaler and ¹/₂ lb.
    Gruyère cheese
Rub a heavy sauce pan with: A clove of garlic
Put into the pan: 2 cups dry white wine

While this is heating uncovered, over moderately high heat,
pour into a cup: 3 tablespoons Kirsch

This is the classic flavoring, although one of the other
dry liqueurs may be used. (Whatever kind of wine, it must
be a dry white wine. Although Kirsch is de rigueur, you may
substitute a nonsweet liqueur like slivovitz, a cognac or
applejack.) Stir into the Kirsch until well dissolved:

1 teaspoon cornstarch

By this time the wine will begin to show small foamy
bubbles over its surface. When it is almost covered with this
fine foam but it is not yet boiling, add the coarsely shredded
cheese gradually, stirring constantly. Keep the heat high but
do not let the fondue boil. Continue to add the cheese until
you can feel a very slight resistance to the spoon as you stir.
Then, still stirring vigorously, add the Kirsch and cornstarch
mixture. Continue to cook until the fondue begins to
thicken.

Add to taste: Nutmeg, white pepper or paprika

Quickly transfer it to a heatproof heavy pan, which can

be placed over an alcohol lamp or chafing dish, or transfer it to an electric skillet adjusted to low heat. After this transferral the cooking continues on low heat and the guests take over. . . .

Note: If there is no white wine to be had, the Bombshell substitutes champagne.

JOSEPHINE'S BONBONS

(She plans to break in the oven with this one)

1 cup butter
1½ cups confectioner's sugar
1 egg
1 teaspoon vanilla extract
1 teaspoon almond extract
2½ cups flour
1 teaspoon baking soda
1 teaspoon cream of tartar

Mix butter and sugar thoroughly. Beat in egg and extracts. Add dry ingredients. Chill for 1 hour. Shape into small balls and place on greased cookie sheet. Optional: press a blanched almond into the center of each. Bake at 375 degrees for ten minutes or so.

SWEDISH MEATBALLS

As cooking is required, the Bombshell asks someone to bring these.

MARILYN MONROE'S DIET PLAN

Breakfast

8:00 A.M.   Orange juice or stewed prunes
             Cereal, well cooked
             Toast (white), 2 slices, crisp, with butter
             Milk or weak cocoa, 1 cup
10:00 A.M.   Milk, 1 cup, and 1 cracker

Lunch or Supper

1:00 P.M.   CHOICE OF:
             Egg, 1 (boiled, poached, shirred or
                 scrambled)
             or cottage cheese, 2 tablespoons

             CHOICE OF:
             Potato, 1, baked or mashed
             or spaghetti, boiled with tomato or butter
                 (no cheese)
             or noodles, $\frac{1}{2}$ cup (boiled), add milk (no
                 cheese)
             Toast or bread (white), stale, 1 slice, with
                 butter
             Jell-O or cooked fruit
3:30 P.M.   Milk, 1 cup, and 1 cracker

Dinner

6:30 P.M.   CHOICE OF:
             Lean beef (boil, broil or roast)
             or chicken
             or lamb chop
             or sweetbread
             or fish

or chicken liver
Potato, 1 (any way but fried)

CHOICE OF:
½ cup tomatoes, beets, carrots, spinach,
    string beans or peas, pureed or strained
Bread (white), 1 slice with butter
Dessert: junket, custard, tapioca pudding or
    rice pudding or baked apple

11:00 P.M.   Eggnog

Beverages

It's not just the bubbles. Like the Bombshell, champagne knows how to make an entrance. Heads turn when it's opened and there's always a little nervous tension. Will the cork break a crystal chandelier or bowl someone over? Will the cup overflow? Dangerously effervescent, champagne, French only, is clearly the favorite drink of the Bombshell. Sparkling, exclusive and frothing with foam—the Bombshell has even been known to take baths in it.[1] Why shouldn't she? Venus was born of the foam of the sea.

When it comes to champagne, no occasion is too small. In fact, no occasion is necessary. A new pair of shoes, a new nail polish, a friend's poem being published, a mourning dove landing on the windowsill—she toasts them all. The Bombshell has been known to order it for a pick-me-up when she feels a little fatigued.[2]

1 Jayne Mansfield bathed in pink champagne twice a week.

2 Brigitte Bardot called for a bottle of champagne while being interviewed for *The New York Times*. "It's the one thing that gives me some zest when I feel tired," she said.

To the Bombshell, champagne goes with any food from potato chips (*The Seven Year Itch*) to hot dogs (*How to Marry a Millionaire*).

As for other drinks, each has a distinct connotation and place. When the Bombshell tries to be grown up, say, a business meeting, she goes for a classic martini. Never a twist, she wants the olive. A somber meeting with a journalist, writer or poet calls for a moody gin and tonic. She'll have a pink lady below the Mason–Dixon line, especially in pink hotels and if her outfit is either pink or cream or off-white chiffon, never with a black cocktail dress. She likes chardonnay in a bathing suit unless she's Mediterranean, in which case she'll have red. The Bombshell will also celebrate with sangria or a margarita when in Mexico, Panama, Spain, Cuba or South America. She knows how to go native and lighten up. She would never order a Manhattan, but she'll pluck the maraschino cherry out of yours.

The Bombshell doesn't like things men drink.[3] Scotch, bourbon, especially beer unless it's indigenous. She has an innate disdain for anything new and pretentious like cosmopolitans, and things have to be pretty bad for a Bombshell to order a Bloody Mary—too blowsy, lushy and depressed. Bombshells love to have a bottle of mineral water for the table, with gas. Bombshells also drink Coke.

---

3 Unless she's freshening up in a hurry and gargles with something from the nearest decanter, i.e., Elizabeth Taylor in *Butterfield 8*.

BOMBSHELL EXERCISE

Most Bombshell exercise can be done on the telephone—leg extensions, calf lifts on a book, and arm exercises with three-pound weights, a must before going out in a strapless gown. Although they may participate, Bombshells do not feel competitive in the sporting arena; they are more interested in putting on the outfit and getting into the spirit of things. Occasionally Bombshells enlist personal trainers or, in the case of Dorothy Dandridge, a physical culturist for balance, poise and inward harmony. Jean Harlow played golf and liked to try out new pools. Marilyn Monroe had a bench press and free weights and also flirted with yoga. Bombshells are famous for dabbling in sports—swimming, horseback riding, badminton, exercise class, yoga, weight lifting, leisurely bicycle rides, tennis, running and miniature golf. In that order.

Bombshell Vacations

The Bombshell generally vacations wherever someone takes her. She does, however, have favorite places, many she's dreamed of visiting since childhood. These are generally places she's seen on luggage stickers, in movies, and read about in books, places her heroines summered, suffered, sashayed and loved. She prefers glamorous, Old World hotels and resorts and has a weakness for any place pink: Bermuda for its pink sand, Florida for pink hotels, any place with flamingos, islands famous for pink coral and a motel near a monastery in southern California she read about in a tour guide and plans to stay in for at least one night, called Tickled Pink.

The Bombshell also visits American landmarks such as the Lincoln Memorial in Washington, D.C., the Tomb of the Unknown Soldier in Arlington, Virginia, the Liberty Bell in Philadelphia, the observation deck of the Empire State Building (she reads all about the Seven Wonders of the World in the lobby), Old Faithful at Yellowstone National Park and the Grand Canyon.

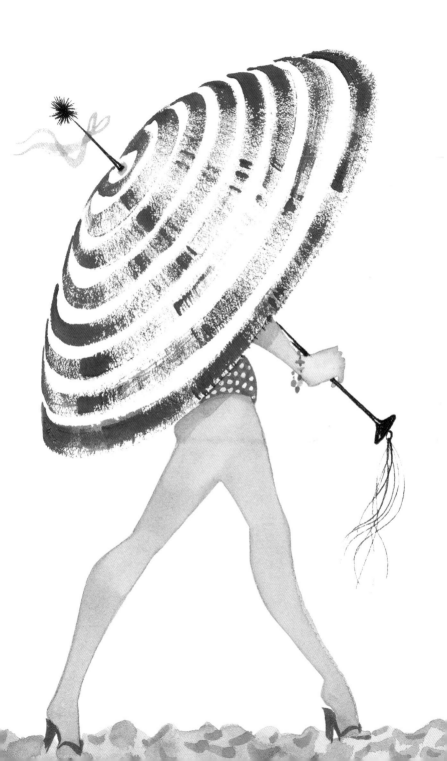

The Bombshell has high expectations about childhood fantasies. If a Bombshell arrives at her destination and finds it shabbier, less glamorous than she'd imagined, she will do her best to find the highlights, to see only what's charming and find beauty even in the tarnish. Of a threadbare velvet chair in a European hotel, she might say, "Why look, I bet thousands of wonderful French books were read here in this chair. Probably Balzac." A worn desk could indicate that love letters were written there. Those ring marks could only be caused by champagne.

It is a well-known fact that the Bombshell likes Hawaii, Niagara Falls, Paris, Monte Carlo, Nice, Cannes, the island of Capri, Bimini, Palm Springs, Lake Tahoe, Venice and Rome. The skiing Bombshell adores the French or Swiss Alps and Vermont if she saw *White Christmas*. The Bombshell may slum it for a romantic weekend in the Poconos but she never does Club Med. Needless to say, she is not fond of camping or any activity that requires swathing on repellent, and has never owned a sleeping bag. The Bombshell believes it's not truly a vacation if you can't get room service, or at the very least, ice from that machine down the hall.

In Los Angeles she adores the bungalows at the old-fashioned Beverly Hills Hotel and the privacy of the Bel Air Hotel, though she'd also be happy to check in at the Chateau Marmont which makes her feel a little like she's in Europe. In southern California the Bombshell likes the Hotel del Coronado, for sentimental, *Some Like It Hot* reasons.

In New York, unless she's feeling low profile, the Bombshell prefers the Plaza Hotel over the Algonquin, but only because she finds Dorothy Parker so sad. She also stays at the Carlyle Hotel, the St. Regis, the Sherry Netherland Hotel and the Waldorf-Astoria.

Landmark Hotels

Hotel du Cap d' Antibes in Cannes. The Bombshell loves the pool that appears to disappear into the sea. She never knows who she'll run into. Rita Hayworth, Sophia Loren, Frank Sinatra, Patricia Arquette, Elizabeth Taylor and Dorothy Dandridge stayed here.

Skyline Brock Hotel. Built in 1929 and overlooking Niagara Falls. The Bombshell knows the blue and pink lights illuminating the falls are tacky and the rooms, save the balconies, are comfortable but nothing special. She likes it anyway.

Cal-Neva Resort, nicknamed "Lady of the Lake," in the Sierra Mountains overlooking Lake Tahoe. The Bombshell has a weakness for anything involving Frank Sinatra, a one-time owner.

The Ahwahnee in Yosemite. Built in 1927 and deemed an architectural wonder, with its 23-foot stained glass windows in the Great Lounge and a majestic mountain view. The Bombshell feels a sense of reverence here.

The Breakers in Palm Beach. That very *La Dolce Vita* fountain out front is her favorite thing. The Bombshell loves a healthy dose of over-the-top Italian Renaissance and the Breakers has been serving it up since it was remodeled in 1926.

The Madonna Inn. She pulled right up when she saw a plethora of pink while driving through San Luis Obispo, California, on the way to Hearst Castle. Her favorite rooms are: Cloud Nine, Fleur-de-lis, Love Nest, Romance and Sugar & Spice.

Hotel Punta Tragara overhanging the Mediterranean Sea in Capri, conceived by Le Corbusier. The Bombshell can't resist a hotel designed by a French architect with a name that sounds like a fancy liqueur.

Vacations a Bombshell Never Takes

Hunting safaris in Africa. (In the documentary *Champagne Safari*, Rita Hayworth was meant to meet her husband Prince Aly Khan on a hunting trip safari. She was a no show.)

Group tours on a motor coach.

Estates that allow fox hunts. If she gets there and finds out animals are hunted, she leaves immediately.

Bed and Breakfasts. The Bombshell thinks, Who are these people? Why am I in their house?

THE LUGGAGE DEPARTMENT

All the clichés are true. A Bombshell en route is ready for anything and has the luggage to prove it. Even a just-moved-in Bombshell with no furniture will have enough luggage to, say, sit on or use as a coffee table.

A Bombshell doesn't know the meaning of traveling light. That mini Louis Vuitton suitcase she's wheeled off the plane is just the beginning. Wheels are not the first consideration of the Bombshell when selecting luggage. She goes for looks, matching pieces: suitcases in several sizes, a vanity and trunk. In addition to Louis Vuitton, the Bombshell favors classic luggage, the kind you can sit on, in pale ivory or tan with dark brown or black leather trim. Occasionally the Bombshell goes for a color to match her lipstick. Marilyn Monroe had a set made in leather-trimmed red canvas by T. Anthony. The Bombshell does not own duffel bags, anything in hard-shell plastic, tapestry or nylon.

The Bombshell travels with what might seem an excessive amount of luggage, not because she is a prima donna, rather she has no idea what may happen and has brought everything. Because packing is always left to the last minute—indeed, the whole trip may be last minute—Bombshell packing rarely involves folding or rolling. The Bombshell is a sentimental packer. Climate is rarely an issue. Who cares if it's thirty below where she's going? She feels so happy in that backless red lamé. Surely there'll be an occasion for that.

All of life counts to the Bombshell, coming and going, boarding, disembarking. You never know who's looking. Most importantly, she wants to feel good about herself. Needless to say, Bombshells always travel in style. While traveling, she will brush her teeth, give herself a facial in the bathroom, apply lotion where needed, spritz on perfume. She knows that the best way to arrive looking well rested is to drink plenty of bottled water—she swears by Fiji—but has been known to slip in a little champagne. She doesn't believe in jet lag; therefore, it doesn't show. All Bombshells throw their coats over their shoulders, never put their arms through, when stepping out of the plane, train or cruiseship.

The Bombshell will carry some of her own luggage—her makeup bag for instance, that mesh bag the dog goes in and possibly the aforementioned Louis Vuitton. Otherwise, luggage throws off her entrance. Sky caps and fellow travelers are quick to heave her luggage onto one of those rolling luggage racks. How could she possibly be expected to do it in those shoes?

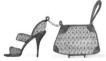

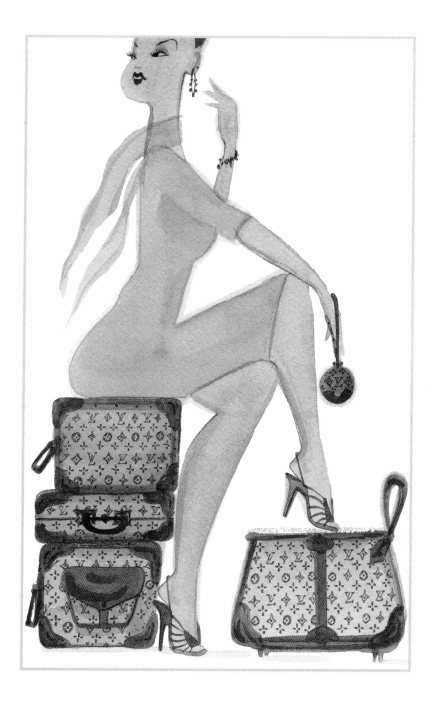

BOMBSHELL TRANSPORTATION

The Bombshell adores chauffeured sedans, taciturn taxi drivers and yachts, but she is happiest when she is in control behind the wheel of something fast and convertible. She favors 1955 Thunderbirds, black or white; 1950 Pontiac convertibles; Cadillacs, white, pink or black; Jaguars; Rolls-Royces and Lincoln Continentals in white, pink and red. If she's not driving, she's happy to be picked up in dark blue. She also likes those little red sport cars. This is not to say she would turn down a ride on a Vespa. Or a Jeep. The Bombshell gets a kick out of life and if her date shows up with say, a Gremlin, she'll see the beauty in it ("How seventies!").

Bombshells have been known to drive without a license and frequently have traffic violations.

The Bombshell also appreciates Shetland pony rides and prefers to ride sidesaddle.

BOMBSHELL WILDLIFE

When it comes to animals, nothing is out of the question. Two wings, one wing, four legs, six legs, the Bombshell loves them all. The Bombshell has empathized with animals all of her life[1] and is particularly drawn to the broken, the abandoned,[2] the doomed.[3]

Kim Novak had a pet fly. "I'll never forget that fly," she said. "My mother swatted him and one of his wings came off, but he didn't die. I cried over him and I kept him for weeks, feeding him sugar."

While the Bombshell sets boundaries for humans, animals have carte blanche; Jayne Mansfield's white poodle

---

1 As a child, Kim Novak put up a sign on her house that read: BRING SICK AND STRAY PETS HERE.

2 A newspaper reported that "No fewer than 60 cats, though, have found refuge in Miss Bardot's own home in St. Tropez—with fifteen dogs, sheep, goats, a horse, a mare and a donkey."

3 Jayne Mansfield claimed that when she worked for a vet, she brought home animals that were about to be put to sleep.

takes a bubble bath with her in *Will Success Spoil Rock Hunter?*

Kim Novak had the door of her house built to accommodate even the largest of her pets, which ranged from llamas to horses to raccoons, so they could wander in and out freely. "This way they realize that you respect them and they respect you," she said. "If you only see your horse when you go out to ride, you don't know your horse." She also gave her raccoon run of the house. "He goes into my refrigerator, gets something to eat, and always leaves the door open," she said. "He even goes into the bathroom, turns on the water, takes a shower, then climbs up on the bed and stretches out."

Legend has it that when Marilyn Monroe heard a calf mooing in the rain she wanted to bring it into the living room so it could dry off. She thought the farmer had forgotten it, but husband-at-the-time Jim Dougherty was not amused.

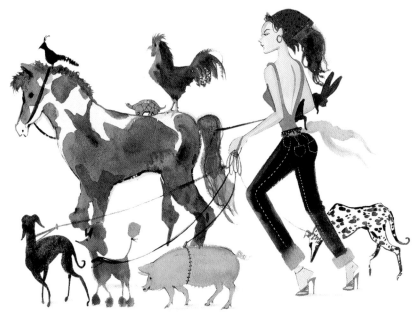

The Bombshell in film has been known to release small birds from cages in the streets of Marseilles, turn on a fire hydrant for a thirsty puppy—of course she ends up taking the puppy home[4]—throw the ultimate throw-herself-on-the-ground-fit to save the life of a baby pig,[5] save a parrot from a jail cell,[6] and there's no way a Bombshell will carry on with a man who is roping wild mustangs for dog food.[7]

Brigitte Bardot has been an animal activist since 1962 and created the Brigitte Bardot Foundation in 1986. According to her website, its ambition is "to be at the heart of the fight for animal rights . . . interven[ing] anywhere in the world where there is mistreatment and cruelty towards animals."

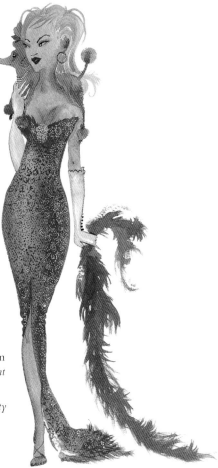

"I gave my beauty and my youth to men," she said in a 1987 *New York Times* interview, "and now I am giving my wisdom and experience, the best of me, to animals."

4 Josephine Baker in *Zouzou*.

5 Brigitte Bardot, while on the lam in the Roger Vadim film *The Night Heaven Fell*.

6 Brigitte Bardot in *That Naughty Girl*.

7 Marilyn Monroe in *The Misfits*.

Bombshells, even when apparel shopping, are easily sidetracked when it comes to animals. The famed celebrity columnist Sidney Skolsky once wrote of Lana Turner: "She is fond of animals, especially dogs. She once went to Beverly Hills to buy a pair of stockings and came back with a full-grown Great Dane instead."

True to her contradictory nature, the Bombshell also views animals as decorative. She has been known to walk ocelots on Hollywood Boulevard (Jayne Mansfield), cheetahs on the Champs-Elysees (Josephine Baker) and dye her standard poodle to match her outfits, from blue to polka dots (Jayne Mansfield in *Will Success Spoil Rock Hunter?*). There is a famous Paul Schumach photograph of Jayne Mansfield holding two Chihuahuas, one in her lap and the other between her breasts as if it were a brooch.

No one can explain why Bombshells attend bullfights and have wild affairs with matadors. They are divided on Hemingway. It's a love-him (Ava Gardner) or hate-him (Marilyn Monroe) kind of thing. Nor can anyone explain why a Bombshell (Kim Novak) gives a pet a bearskin rug upon which to sleep. These are inconsistencies granted to the Bombshell. There are no absolute rules.

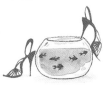

IV

Bombshell Pursuits & Ideals

BOMBSHELL ART

The Bombshell, much to everyone's surprise, adores Jackson Pollock. She likes him in the way she cares about injured pit bulls, wounded parrots, foster children and juvenile delinquents. She loves that he danced in the barn in black jeans, loafers and T-shirt while dripping paint on canvases that covered the floor. To the Bombshell, Jackson Pollock is the James Dean of the art world. Dangerous, from the Wild West, hard-living, and dead at the height of his career from a car accident, he's as glamorous and tragic as it gets.

She likes him even more than the Impressionists, whom she cannot help but love because they are soothing, especially Renoir, whose brush strokes seem sugar-spun, like cotton candy and almost as much as Botticelli's *Birth of Venus*. She is suspicious of Picasso but adores him all the same. His blue and rose period paintings tug at her heart the way Keane paintings of children and animals with big eyes do. Mandolins and harlequins get to her. After all, if it's good enough for Frank Sinatra to have a harlequin motif on an album cover, it must be poignantly poetic.

The Bombshell does not want to be challenged by art. She does not favor violence, ugliness, poverty, toil. Melancholy she understands and she always falls for a good story. This makes Vincent van Gogh one of her favorites. Though not wooed by the coarseness of his portraits, those flowers and landscapes have more personality then some of the men she's dated. The Bombshell is sure that if she'd been there, somehow, van Gogh's paintings would have sold. In the film *Panic Button*, Jayne Mansfield helps a starving artist by inviting gentlemen to her "studio" and selling his work as her own.

The Bombshell loves Rubens for his full-bodied appreciation of women and Georgia O'Keeffe for her full-bodied appreciation of flowers. She could live without the cow skulls. A Bombshell only likes Andy Warhol if it's a picture of her.

The Bombshell's Twenty Favorite Works of Art

1 *Odalisque* by Jean-Auguste-Dominique Ingres
2 *The Bather* by Jean-Auguste-Dominique Ingres
3 *Sunflowers* by Vincent van Gogh
4 *Starry Night* by Vincent van Gogh
5 *Waterlilies* by Claude Monet
6 *The Bar at the Folies-Bergère* by Édouard Manet
7 *The Birth of Venus* by Sandro Botticelli
8 *The Medici Venus* by an unknown Hellenistic sculptor
9 *Venus de Milo* by an unknown Hellenistic sculptor
10 *The Nude Maja* by Francisco de Goya
11 *Lavender Mist* by Jackson Pollock
12 *The Kiss* by Auguste Rodin

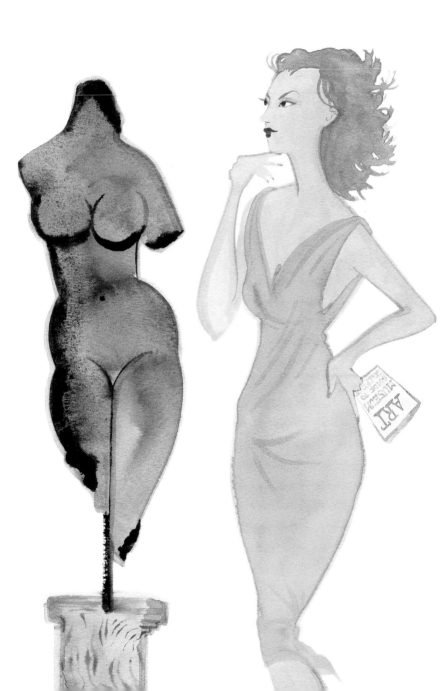

13 *The Kiss* by Gustav Klimt
14 *David* by Michelangelo
15 *The Three Graces* by Raphael
16 *The Swing* by Jean-Honoré Fragonard
17 *The Saltimbanques* and most of the blue period paintings by Pablo Picasso
18 *Girl with a Pearl Earring* by Johannes Vermeer
19 *Déjeuner sur l'Herbe* by Édouard Manet
20 *Mona Lisa* by Leonardo da Vinci

Art and Artists a Bombshell Does Not Like

Francis Bacon
Hieronymus Bosch
Lucian Freud
German Expressionists
Frida Kahlo
Henri de Toulouse-Lautrec
Medieval painting and sculpture
Edvard Munch
Louise Nevelson (All that grotesque black and those awful eyelashes.)
Philip Perlstein
Egon Schiele
Frank Stella (A black dress she understands, but a painting??)
Surrealists

BOMBSHELL HOBBIES

"What good is it just to be pretty?" says Kim Novak as Madge in *Picnic*. "Maybe I get tired of only being looked at."

In her constant quest to improve, the Bombshell dabbles in the arts and letters. Life drawing, literature courses, art appreciation. She takes poetry workshops, acting classes, singing, dance—tango to tap to ballet—and French. She also takes guitar lessons and photography. She intends to take a cooking class someday.

In a 1950s interview, Dorothy Dandridge named psychology as her favorite study because it "not only helps her to understand other people but herself as well." She listed her other hobbies as interior decorating, collecting records, horseback riding and cooking.

BOMBSHELL GAMES

Bombshells cheat at card games. Go fish, hearts, gin rummy, canasta, pinochle and cribbage. They admit this, even Sophia Loren. Most people think it's charming if money's not involved. If the above-mentioned card games are played at her home, there will be red pistachios and peanut M & Ms or nonpareils in a crystal candy dish on the card table, which will be of the folding variety.

The Bombshell adores parlor games. Charades is her favorite. She likes to have the novelist and playwright on her side; an actor will do in a pinch. The Bombshell prefers Candyland to Monopoly, checkers to chess, Scrabble to Trivial Pursuit. She has her own internal dictionary with a voluptuous range of exotic words not found in any standard dictionary. Five consonants, two of them *x*'s? No problem.

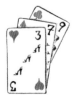

BOMBSHELL HUSBANDS

The Bombshell gets married. That is not to say that the Bombshell has not shacked up, but it's not her style. She wants respect. Commitment. The ring.

"I hate to be alone," Jane Russell told the *New York Sunday News*. "I was born married. I need a man at my side constantly." The Bombshell is so committed to the idea of forever that she is willing to gamble on love again and again and again.

The man a Bombshell marries does not have to be loaded or able to advance her career—but he is rarely the guy next door.[1] Brigitte Bardot once said she didn't like rich men. "They think they can buy everything, including me."

The Bombshell husband has to be good at something: have a title, talent, or be heroic. A Bombshell may say her vows to a millionaire playboy, but she's more likely to fall for an actor (Elizabeth Taylor and Richard Burton, Patricia

---

1 Elizabeth Taylor tried it with husband number eight, construction worker Larry Fortensky.

Arquette and Nicolas Cage), an American hero (Marilyn Monroe and Joe DiMaggio), a prince (Rita Hayworth and Aly Khan), Mr. Universe (Jayne Mansfield and Mickey Hargitay), a crooner (Ava Gardner and Frank Sinatra), a bandleader (Lana Turner/Ava Gardner and Artie Shaw), or she might just settle down with a veterinarian, who, in the eyes of a Bombshell, is the ultimate hero. Kim Novak did. Bombshells also like to be muses. They marry playwrights (Marilyn Monroe and Arthur Miller), directors (Rita Hayworth and Orson Welles), or anyone in the arts they feel they can inspire.

HOW A BOMBSHELL
AMUSES A MAN

Let it be known that the Bombshell works on a subconscious level and never tries to be amusing. To men, or anyone. We may not be immune to her tight sweater or high heels, but this is not how she puts us in her thrall. There are four Bombshell behaviors that reel you in.

Laughter

The Bombshell laughs. Never at anyone, unless, of course, it's herself. She is perpetually amused and delighted, never stingy with her response. The Bombshell makes people feel amusing.

Kim Novak once said, "The best way to lose a man is to make too many jokes at his expense. Most men are more vain than any female. They think everything they say is funny. Pretty soon, if you play up to his vanity, he gets to figuring out you might be a wonderful person to have around the rest of his life."

There are many varieties of Bombshell laughter: the surprised, mewlike exhale of Jayne Mansfield, the breathy giggle of Marilyn Monroe, the baby laugh of Patricia Arquette, the earthy, warm laugh of Sophia Loren emanating from the solar plexus. The Bombshell never snorts, honks, roars, pounds the table or slaps her thigh. The Bombshell laugh is not flat, monotone, nasal or staccato. Bombshells also smile frequently.

Leaning

The Bombshell leans into conversation. She gets intimate. Takes it all in. She's not afraid of invading your personal space or letting you invade hers. The Bombshell is literally on the edge of her seat.

Listening

The Bombshell is notorious for her candor. She admits everything. She is not, however, in the habit of blurting out maudlin details or offering unsolicited testimonials. The Bombshell is more interested in hearing your story. She asks questions. Intelligent questions. Whether it's the story of your childhood, the latest NFL trade, or the poetry of Carl Sandburg, she's all yours.

Looking

The Bombshell makes eye contact. Once she is engaged in conversation, she gives you 100 percent of her attention. She does not scan the room to see who is watching, who just left or what's on the hors d'oeuvres tray.

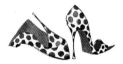

V

Bombshell Miscellanea

The Bombshell's
Ten Favorite Movies

1 *It's a Wonderful Life*
2 *Bambi* (A box of Kleenex is needed for this one. She loves it anyway.)
3 *Tarzan and His Mate* (The 1934 version with Johnny Weissmuller and Maureen O'Sullivan. A strong, heroic man and a playful chimp. Bombshell heaven.)
4 *Hamlet* with Laurence Olivier
5 *Mr. Hulot's Holiday*
6 *Romeo and Juliet* (The one made in 1936 starring Leslie Howard and Norma Shearer.)
7 *Gone With the Wind*
8 Cecil B. DeMille's *Cleopatra*
9 *A Little Princess* (She loves a rags-to-riches story. She also loves the monkey.)
10 *The Hunchback of Notre Dame* (with Charles Laughton and Maureen O'Hara.)

THE BOMBSHELL ZODIAC

The Aries Bombshell

Aries says Bombshell with a big bang. She is not at all shy, but that does not mean she isn't shamelessly feminine. It's just that her other qualities are the first thing you notice. Decisive, impulsive, spontaneous, independent, generous, Aries is ruled by Mars, the planet of action. The Aries Bombshell is not afraid to volunteer, roll up her sleeves, jump right in. The Aries Bombshell might decide, suddenly, to paint her bedroom wall pink and do it that weekend. Herself. She is better at initiating projects than finishing them and it is good for her to have a Capricorn or Taurus around, even though she finds them a bit sluggish. The Aries Bombshell is restless and is not the desk-job type. It is commonly believed that red is the favorite color of the Aries Bombshell, when in fact she often prefers red's paler cousin, pink. Ruby pink, ice pink, peony pink; adding a little white to crimson in no way dilutes the Aries flame.

The Taurus Bombshell

The Taurus is generally too sensible and earthy to be a Bombshell. Yet no other sign can be as formidable when she succumbs to the sensual traits of her ruling planet, Venus. The Taurus Bombshell is gifted with a beautiful voice; deep and sultry, it's a veritable caress. Whether she is gamine or overflowing with curves, she has grace, humor and poise. Anita Loos, author of *Gentlemen Prefer Blondes,* was a Taurus. So was Liberace. More than any other sign, the Taurus Bombshell knows how to create a lush, opulent atmosphere; no uncomfortable chairs in her home and never harsh lights.

The Taurus Bombshell has a weakness for bonbons and all things chocolate. She adores cream sauces, fine wines, leisurely dinners. She always knows what cognac or champagne to order, but she holds back her opinion if someone less savvy is ordering. She likes to take her time, whether it's getting ready to go out or writing a thank-you note—never rush the Taurus Bombshell. She appreciates material expressions of love (emeralds, sapphires, etc.), particularly if they are heirlooms. She prefers fabrics with substance such as cashmere, shantung and suede and favors dusty pastels, especially greens, pink, violet, copper and fawn.

The Gemini Bombshell

Easily distracted, Gemini is the most flirtatious of the sun signs. She may have a fragile, flickering hummingbird quality, but her magnetism can be felt from across the room. Of all the Bombshells of the zodiac, the Gemini is the friendliest, the most likely to have excess charisma. She empathizes with anything helpless and it is best not to relay tragic animal stories unless you plan to ruin her day.

The Gemini Bombshell is not big on discipline and likes to have a coach, or a few, since she'll be working on several things simultaneously. Acting lessons, singing lessons, yoga classes, anything with a schedule helps. The Gemini Bombshell loves all colors, and being bubbly, wears polka dots with greater aplomb than any other sign. Yellow—from chrysanthemum to ivory—is favored by the Gemini Bombshell.

The Cancer Bombshell

The Bombshell is not known for her prowess in the kitchen, and the Cancer Bombshell is no exception. She does, however, like to entertain and is the Bombshell most likely to have actually used her oven. The Cancer is the homebody of the zodiac; home is where she retreats when she needs to recharge, regroup, take cover. She may also bring home sick animals and invite over depressed girlfriends, make them tea and order in Chinese. And if a man falls into her lair, forget about it. (You can be sure there's a bottle of Dom Pérignon in the refrigerator.)

The Cancer Bombshell is likely to be late, not because she is fixing her hair but because she might notice that the crystal needs rearranging or because she suddenly gets it into her head that the Wedgwood china would really look better on that other shelf.

She may appear buoyant and outgoing, but she is deeply sensitive and easily wounded. If you hurt her feelings it may take forever for her to let you know.

This Bombshell has an extensive collection of attire that is exclusively for lounging. Billowing palazzo pants, kaftans, silk pajamas in watery blues, lavenders, greens. She feels most herself in slippery fabrics and is luminous in plunging silver, oyster and grey. Dangling pearl earrings suit her even better than diamonds.

The Leo Bombshell

The Leo Bombshell likes to run her own show, and when making public appearances, tucks her vulnerability into her underpinnings. She can be quite daring (think Amelia Earhart), and is at her best when she is the center of attention.

Her biggest weakness, in fact, is that she adores being in the spotlight—precisely why she is so lovable. As the sign ruled by the sun, she always manages to stand where the light is most flattering. She has a voluptuous ego and has been known to frighten off less confident men with her excess of va-va-voom. She expects roses and flattery but it has to be sincere. She can always tell.

Dignified drama best describes her style. Majestic velvets in royal blue, burgundy, scarlet, purple, gold and black with plunging backs or necklines, feline prints of every kind, shimmering silk gowns and blouses in light-catching oyster, champagne and ivory live up to her exuberance. She can carry off exotic and tropical prints but is rarely seen in demure flowers. There is no green in the Leo Bombshell wardrobe other than emeralds. She bears no malice or jealousy and is the kind of woman who will happily share her perfume and beauty secrets. Be careful what you admire when it comes to the Leo Bombshell. She is likely to give you whatever it is, or send you one later.

The Virgo Bombshell

Cool and mysterious, the Virgo Bombshell has a hide-and-go-seek air about her. She may be maddeningly elusive, and it is not always easy to be sure of her affections. There is something modest and pure about her, even when she is wearing a cut-to-there neckline. Mercurial hues suit the Virgo Bombshell. She can carry off virginal white eyelet dresses—fitted, of course—as well as fitted suits in steely blue and svelte sleeveless dresses in silver and deep grey. She likes clean, ethereal perfumes such as Chanel No. 19, and she will always have a perfect manicure. Every hair is in place on the Virgo Bombshell; even if it's an extravagant mess, you can be sure she's planned it that way. Virgo Bombshells do not allow for chance when it comes to appearances. When the Virgo Bombshell is in a casual mood, she favors a crisp cotton bra that peeps out ingeniously from under a tailored white shirt, probably worn with slim blue slacks or Capri pants. When she's at the beach or really roughing it, she might throw on a white peasant blouse and, after a martini or two, allow it to fall off her shoulders and reveal more than her well-defined clavicles.

The Libra Bombshell

Ruled by the planet Venus, Libra is the ultimate love goddess, the most charming of all the signs. This is not something cultivated. She was born this way. The Libra Bombshell loves beauty, harmony and chocolates and can't bear to be alone. Surprisingly, she has some domestic skill when it comes to decorating. This will manifest primarily in the bedroom. She may sew her own curtains from Alençon lace she found in Paris, or make her own lampshades. She will also take sleeves off dresses, nip in waists, cut off collars. Her clothing is always on the snug and sexy side. And she loves pink. No one is more effusive than the Libra Bombshell when she receives a gift, even if she hates it. *Graciousness* is the operative word.

The Libra Bombshell has an undeserved reputation for laziness when the truth is she simply understands the art of relaxation more than any other sign. Bubble baths, room sprays, fragrant oils, pillows, mood lighting, music, she excels at them all. While other signs might bring soup or hot tea to a friend who is under the weather, the Libra's idea of healing involves scented candles and a facial.

The Libra Bombshell has a pinch of diva and it is rare to find one who does not like to sing, even if she is alone.

The Scorpio Bombshell

If the Scorpio Bombshell had to be summed up in one word, it would be *intense*. She might be a water sign but there's nothing wishy-washy about her. Red and black are her colors (think long, form-fitting black knits, tight red sweaters) and she is not the type to tinker with pastels and flimsy fabrics. She throws herself into projects with tireless determination and if you tell her she's not right for a part or a job, she'll stare directly into your eyes and convince you otherwise. She is the most bewitching of all Bombshells and seems to have a sixth sense about things. Never lie to the Scorpio Bombshell; she'll see through you like cellophane. She chooses perfumes that are distinctive. No soft florals or powdery Jicky for her. She adores Youth Dew, Tabu, Tabac Blond, Gardenia Passion. At her most kittenish, Shalimar. (She loves spice.)

There's something awe inspiring about the Scorpio Bombshell gait. Her derrière has a delightful wiggle, and seems to be propelled by an invisible force—perhaps her scorpion tail. Is she vindictive like the astrology books say she is? Not the Scorpio Bombshell. She rises above most injury with haughty majesty—she'll let karma do its thing—

but it should be noted that no other Bombshell can compete with her tantrum. A spurned Scorpio Bombshell leaves no stemware unscathed.

Her stone is opal but she appreciates carnelian and rubies.

The Sagittarius Bombshell

She is the Bombshell most likely to take up flying, sky diving, scuba diving, anything with a little risk and adventure. Fresh, open and frank, she is the most restless Bombshell in the zodiac, the least materialistic, and the most athletic. She may have marabou mules (next to the riding boots) in the back of her closet, but she'll spend more time picking out alluring exercise ensembles than ballgowns—she likes these in sleek, clingy, no-frills silhouettes—and is more inclined to go swing dancing or cycling than take a calligraphy course.

She will be more charmed by a beautiful poem than flowers (she may secretly write poetry herself, kept in a journal by her bed), and more impressed by your record for a 10K race than your 401k.

Her lounging attire includes several white terry cloth robes and one in waffle piqué she bought in Rome.

She is direct and she'll always tell you the truth whether you can bear to hear it or not. Don't tell her any secrets because she is too guileless to remember that she's not supposed to tell.

She is often the life of the party, and her idea of a great evening is attending three cocktail parties in one night and then splashing in a public fountain with that polo player she met at the last one.

The Capricorn Bombshell

No other Bombshell interprets body language more precisely than the Capricorn. She can read volumes into a handshake, a slump, a stride, a look. She is virtually impossible to deceive. Her own body language is provocative and no sign can cross her legs with greater poise.

The Capricorn Bombshell consciously strives to overcome her naturally melancholic nature by smiling and laughing a lot. She has, in fact, an offbeat sense of humor. The Capricorn Bombshell may be giddy one moment and quite serious the next and her sense of style reflects her dual nature. One summer evening she may show up in pale blue chiffon; the following day it's a slim, black gabardine skirt and tan tailored shirt. Her clothing is deceptively conservative; the Capricorn Bombshell wears even the most traditional garb in such a way that it is stylish and provocative (think tight, unbuttoned). That chic little black dress, her favorite, might not have a low neckline, but a pin placed just so could distract an entire room all evening.

She favors tweeds, glen plaids, camel hair and cashmere. The Capricorn Bombshell is the most status-conscious of all the signs. Although she finds it gauche to flash labels, she feels more confident knowing her gown is YSL, her slingbacks Manolo, her trench Burberry. Above all, she appreciates quality. She'd rather have one fabulous cashmere sweater than twenty in mere merino wool.

The Aquarius Bombshell

There is something elusive and a little aloof about the Aquarius Bombshell. There is an electricity about her, something crackling beneath her cool exterior. Unimpressed by traditional, generic offerings like long-stemmed red roses, the Aquarius must be wooed by unconventional gifts. A vintage copy of *Through the Looking Glass* or *The Giant Golden Book of Elves and Fairies,* or a tiny, cute, newfangled camera (she has a weakness for gadgets) is more likely to tickle her fancy. Honest, altruistic, breezy and offbeat—there's never a dull moment with an Aquarian Bombshell. She has a way of shocking people without even trying. She might, for example, wear an evening gown to the beach or show up with a chimp at the Christmas party. She also takes up causes. Her stone is aquamarine; her prints Pucci and paisley; her colors cobalt and electric blue. Nevertheless—she hates being told what to do—she might choose fuchsia just to be contrary.

The Pisces Bombshell

There's depth beneath that serene, calm, sphinxlike exterior. The Pisces Bombshell is the most feminine of all. It is said she has an old soul, but she is the most childlike Bombshell and the one most likely to burst into tears. Old movies, sad stories, they all get to her. The Pisces is the consummate actress; she can identify with just about everyone. She adopts the wounded animal and defends the underdog. She can forgive anyone almost anything, given enough time, and is the sign most likely, next to Gemini and Aquarius, to have pen pals in prison.

Ethereal colors (leafy greens, seafoam, cerulean blue, cobalt blue, lavender) best suit her, though in pale pink and light beige she virtually fades away. Black, too, suits the Pisces and her sense of melodrama and chic. If she's in a highly charged mood, she can carry off red, but it's best for her to stay with dreamy colors that play up her subtle, fairy-like allure. She favors filmy, unsubstantial materials, has an affinity for sequins and owns an extensive collection of kimonos. She is one of the few signs that can carry off flowers, such as daisies (see the white, flower-trimmed dress Elizabeth Taylor wore in *A Place in the Sun*). The Pisces gem is moonstone but she's not opposed to diamonds.

Bombshell Star Signs

Aries	Patricia Arquette, Jayne Mansfield
Taurus	Anita Loos, Ann-Margret
Gemini	Josephine Baker, Marilyn Monroe, Jane Russell
Cancer	Gina Lollobrigida
Leo	Mae West
Virgo	Sophia Loren
Libra	Brigitte Bardot, Rita Hayworth
Scorpio	Dorothy Dandridge, Veronica Lake, Hedy Lamarr
Sagittarius	Kim Basinger, Dorothy Lamour, Marisa Tomei
Capricorn	Ava Gardner
Aquarius	Kim Novak, Lana Turner
Pisces	Drew Barrymore, Jean Harlow, Elizabeth Taylor

THE BOMBSHELL QUIZ

1 You're awakened by the bell while sleeping in the buff.
  You . . .
  a. Think, I'm not expecting company, I need my
     beauty rest.
  b. Ask who it is and throw on an oversized T-shirt
     before answering.
  c. Spritz on perfume, fluff your hair and envelop your-
     self in a sheet before answering.
2 You're feeling blue. You . . .
  a. Put on Frank Sinatra.
  b. Have Veuve Clicquot delivered.
  c. Draw a bubble bath.
3 You're about to purchase a pair of Manolos when the
  woman next to you exclaims, "I have to have those!"
  They are the last pair. You . . .
  a. Hand them over.
  b. Help the poor thing search the shop for what suits
     her better.
  c. Ignore her.

4 You're driving down the highway with a gentleman and see a dog hit by a car. You . . .
   a. Determine to make a donation to the ASPCA.
   b. Report the license plate number to the authorities.
   c. Stop the car and make him scoop up the dog and take it to the vet.

5 You're at work and get a run in your pantyhose. You . . .
   a. Go home ill.
   b. Patch it up with some nail polish.
   c. Peel them off.

6 After a swim at the beach you discover sand in your bikini. You . . .
   a. Slip it off and rinse it in the ocean.
   b. Cultivate a devil-may-care attitude and have a beer on your towel.
   c. Walk the two hundred yards to the showers.

7 You're pulled over on the interstate for speeding. You . . .
   a. Burst into tears and relay a heart-wrenching story.
   b. Show a little leg.
   c. Smile, make eye contact, hand over your license and compliment his boots.

8 You have five hundred dollars to your name. You . . .
   a. Pay your rent on time. After all, a girl needs a roof over her head as much as a diamond necklace needs a jewelry box.
   b. Buy that little dress you've been eyeing and donate the rest to The Dian Fossey Gorilla Fund International.
   c. Call that investment banker and ask him how to invest it.

9 Your idea of breakfast is . . .
   a. Bacon, eggs, toast and orange juice.

   b. Leftover hors d'ouevres.

   c. Champagne and toast.

10 You've invited your latest paramour over for a home-cooked dinner. You . . .

   a. Order in lobster, baked potatoes and corn on the cob from the local gourmet shop and serve it on your own china. He'll never know you didn't rattle those pots and pans.

   b. Put on Frank Sinatra and your favorite dress, flip through all your cookbooks, and decide to serve cocktails instead.

   c. Research his favorite dish and attempt to re-create it.

11 You're introduced to an up-and-coming photographer at a party and he asks you to pose nude. You . . .

   a. Throw your drink in his face.

   b. Tell him you have to lose fifteen pounds first.

   c. Ask, "Black and white or color?"

ANSWERS: 1. c 2. All of the above 3. b 4. c 5. Trick question: Bombshells don't wear pantyhose. 6. a 7. c 8. b 9. Any of the above 10. b 11. c

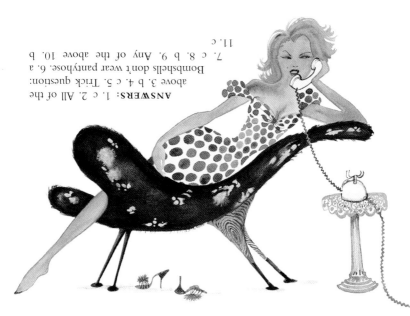

THE WRITERS

Laren Stover's taboo-breaking first novel, *Pluto, Animal Lover* (HarperCollins, 1994), a finalist for the Discover Great New Writers Award, isn't likely to be found on Bombshell bookshelves. A resident of The Writers Room, Laren has received fellowships to Yaddo and Hawthornden Castle and has received the Ludwig Vogelstein Foundation grant for fiction as well as the Dana Award. Her short fiction and poetry have appeared in various literary magazines and her essays have been published in *The New York Times*, German *Vogue* and *The New York Observer*.

Kimberly Forrest was an editor at *W* and *Women's Wear Daily* in Los Angeles and New York where she covered movie premieres and reported on diamonds, moonstones, emeralds, handbags and hats. She now creates color names and concepts for Prescriptives.

Vogue has called **Nicole Burdette** "the Holly Golightly dramatist of New York City." She is a cofounder of the

Naked Angels Theater Company where she has acted and written plays since 1986. She adapted her play, *Chelsea Walls*, for the film *Last Word on Paradise* and has written a screenplay based on the novel *Billy Dead* for Maverick Entertainment. Nicole appeared as Mable in *A River Runs Through It* and most recently in the television series *The Sopranos*. She is a contributing editor to *Bomb* magazine and her fiction has appeared in *Jane* and the *QPB Literary Review*. She teaches writing at The Writers' Voice at the YMCA. Nicole's mother advises stilettos when there is a mouse in the house.

Pop culture savant **Randi Gollin** has written for *MTV News*, *The New York Times*, *Interview*, *Rolling Stone*, *Foodie* and *Seventeen*. She believes that every woman has an inner Bombshell simmering just below the surface.

THE ARTIST

Ruben Toledo has designed mannequins, store windows, award statuettes, scarves and fabrics. He has painted murals, portraits, tiles, album covers and barns and has created witty, incisive illustrations for *L' Uomo Vogue, The New York Times, Harper's Bazaar, Details*, *Paper, Visionaire,* Louis Vuitton and Tiffany. The author of *Style Dictionary* (Abbeville Press), his work has been exhibited at the Metropolitan Museum of Art, the Musée de la Mode et du Textile at the Louvre, and the Museum at the Fashion Institute of Technology. Richard Martin, former curator of the Metropolitan Museum of Art Costume Institute, called Ruben "the greatest fashion illustrator chronicling our time . . . the artist who gives us the vocabulary and the unforgettable images that meld fashion at its most ephemeral and impressionable with style at its most abiding."

Acknowledgments

The writers would like to thank:

Bob Miller for his va-va-voom vision; Jennifer Lang for lavish attention and color in Singapore; Mary Ellen O'Neill for opening the Hyperion door . . .

Christy Fletcher at Carlisle & Co. for patience, passion, razzmatazz under pressure and fine print genius; Lori Applebaum for handling the mundane with voluptuous diplomacy and cheer; Paul Gregory Himmelein for mixing verbal cocktails, poetic musing on art (and just about everything else that concerns this book), sauteeing brussels sprouts and Quarking until dawn; Rick Marin (knight in shining armor) for the horse this book rode in on; Ilene Rosenzweig for high-wattage *NYT* editing and popcorn at midnight; Trip Gabriel for giving the Bombshell stylish, front-page coverage; Carrie Knoblock for adorability and careful sourcing; Craig Nelson for high-heeled inspiration and down-to-earth advice; Liz Dougherty for the polka-dot bikini of prototypes; Alan Kaufman for wise Libran council (a Bombshell adores men who attempt icy walks in patent leather dress shoes). . . .

Marisa Tomei for sashaying up that aisle in her kimono at the Algonquin and giving the Bombshell text authority and curvaceous intelligence; Alan Buchman for old-fashioned showmanship; Glenn O'Brien for making us blonde crazy; Heather Bucha for her smart bomb reading; the Algonquin Hotel for inviting us in; the moms Patricia DiMeo and Shirley Forrest who answered myriad and oddball questions at all hours; Rory Gevis for artful eyelash batting; James Gager for M•A•C-Bombshell ardor; John Demsey for M•A•C-simian simpatico; Ken Miller for last-minute editing (and for the lights on the makeup table); Michael Fabiani for flying in Tabac Blond before it hit Manhattan; Aloysius Lipio for names and numbers that kept us on the scented trail; Robert Gerstner for unraveling perfume mysteries; Andrée Carroon for eggnog at 11:00 and the behind-the-scenes glimpse at Christie's; Ed Arentz for technicolor generosity; Joseph Alfieris for southern hospitality and leggy cover designs; Sara Lee for the ladybug–embellished hideaway (and strong coffee); Sainte Ennis and Monsieur LaFrenier for weekends at the Cran; Robert Vizet for the computer with the personalized screams and breakfast at Tiffany; Lisa Johnson and Valerie Cates for astrology dish; William Calvert for dressing us up; Jennifer Wolinetz for Guerlain stories and ingredients; Katherine Holmes for awakening our senses to Arpège; Valerie Van Galder for outrageous enthusiasm and Isabel Toledo for saying all the right things.

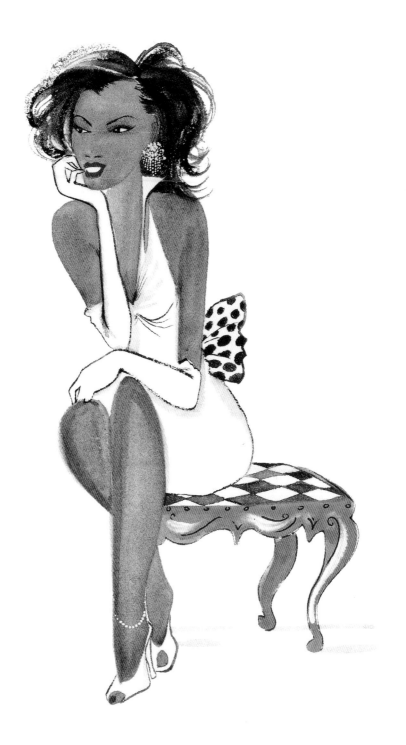

The writers would also like to thank the wildly talented Pauline St. Denis, detail-princess Laura Himmelein, owlish Gary Nargi, Jeff Cooperman for the first bomb, Vredy Lightsman, Yuko de Haan, Stuart de Haan, The Rainbow Room, Susan Hauser, Frankie Foye, Shay, Bari Lynn, Katherine Lantuche for long Bembo proposal hours, Shawn Stewart Ruff (who can tell you why some of the sexiest women are men), Donna Brodie, the Jeanne d'Arc of the Writers Room, Boca Bombshell DeeDee Shullman and Cat-baby.

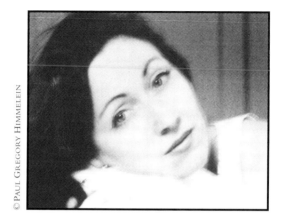

© PAUL GREGORY HIMMELEIN

LAREN STOVER is the author of the novel *Pluto, Animal Lover*. She has been a resident of Yaddo and Hawthornden Castle and received the Ludwig Vogelstein Foundation grant for fiction and the Dana Award. She lives in New York City and can be reached at www.bombshellmanual.com.

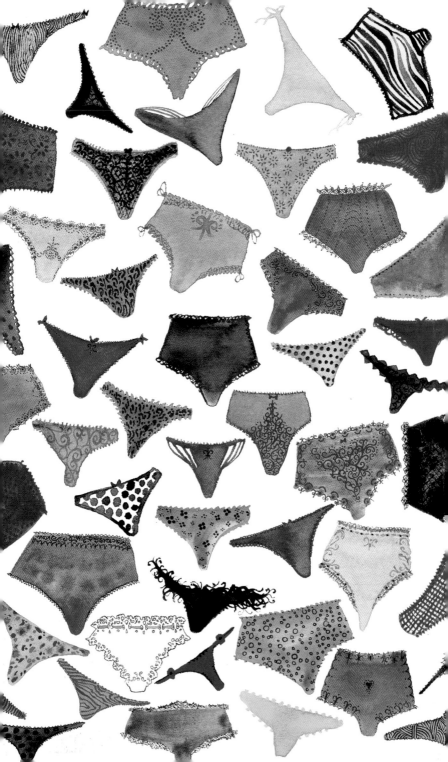